Praise for *How to Create a Vegan World*

"Tobias Leenaert's writings are consistently some of the sharpest and most perceptive material in the animal protection movement's literature. His advice gives activists the tools to play a decisive role in ending the era of industrialized animal exploitation."—**Erik Marcus**, publisher of Vegan.com

"As religious, political, and dietary dogma enjoys a heyday, *How to Create a Vegan World* offers pragmatists a welcome haven. With research supporting his position, the author contends that in valuing both small changes and sweeping ones, we can build, rather than bulldoze, our way to a compassionate and sustainable world."—**Victoria Moran**, author, *Main Street Vegan*, and director, Main Street Vegan Academy

"The animal rights movement has been waiting for a book like this. Tobias Leenaert goes beyond the obvious reasons of why the world should go vegan and provides valuable insights on how to effectively make progress towards that goal. I would highly recommend this book to new and veteran activists dedicated to helping as many animals as they can."—**Nick Cooney**, Vice President of Mercy for Animals, author, *Veganomics* and *Change of Heart*

"Tobias Leenaert has a unique and practical point of view on all things vegan that cuts through the issues like a knife through a firm cake of tofu. He is not afraid to challenge common misconceptions and norms with his penetrating, fact-based reasoning. Always independent and illuminating, we count on activists like Tobias to lead the way towards a vegan world."—**Seth Tibbott**, founder and president, the Tofurky Company

"*How to Create a Vegan World* is a must-read for anyone who wants to maximize their impact to make the world a better place for animals. Tobias Leenaert synthesizes a wealth of research with his own extensive experience as a vegan advocate to present clear arguments and practical tips for effective vegan advocacy. I highly recommend this book!"—**Melanie Joy**, PhD, author, *Why We Love Dogs, Eat Pigs, and Wear Cows*; cofounder and codirector, Center for Effective Vegan Advocacy

"Some animal advocates are content just to be right. Tobias Leenaert doesn't want you to be just right; he wants you to be both right and effective. There's a big difference, and he'll show you what it is."—**Paul Shapiro**, The Humane Society of the United States

"Tobias Leenaert is one of today's most important writers regarding animal issues. Probably his greatest strength is his ability to stay focused on what will actually help animals in the real world. Especially in this time of social media and filtered feeds, it is incredibly easy to focus on what is popular with people who are already vegan. Tobias, however, looks beyond his likes and retweets, and instead stays focused on the bottom line—reaching new people with the message of compassion."—**Matt Ball**, author, *The Accidental Activist*, and coauthor, *The Animal Activist's Handbook*

"If the meat industry had to pick one book they don't want you to read, this would be it."—**Sebastian Joy**, founder and director, ProVeg International

"Big-hearted and level-headed Tobias Leenaert shows us how we need both idealism and pragmatism in the animal rights movement, and that we can make greater, more strategic strides through collaboration, inclusiveness, and meeting people where they're at. Listen to Tobias."—**Jo-Anne McArthur**, photojournalist, author, *We Animals* and *Captive*

"Tobias Leenaert makes a very convincing argument for why a 'food first' approach should be an essential part of the strategic toolbox of the animal advocacy movement. A refreshing, compelling, and ultimately very positive book that should be read by everyone who wants to help animals."—**Bruce Friedrich**, executive director, Good Food Institute

"The single most important book on the subject. With wit, compassion, and humor, Tobias brilliantly combines light-hearted stories with hard-hitting facts, ultimately leaving the reader with a renewed sense of purpose and joy. If you want to master the most effective strategies for reducing societal consumption of animal products, this ultimate guide is for you."—**Brian Kateman**, editor, *The Reducetarian Solution*, and cofounder, the Reducetarian Foundation

"Drawing from the research on successful behavior change as well as his own extensive experience, Tobias Leenaert has created an essential tool for anyone who wants to change the world for animals. *How to Create a Vegan World* is thoughtful, pragmatic, and provocative. It's also packed with useful tips that are likely to make your advocacy more effective than ever."—**Virginia Messina, MPH, RD**, author, *Vegan for Life*, and coauthor, *Even Vegans Die*

"Tobias Leenaert doesn't want to be right but applies a pragmatic approach to create a big societal transition. He does this with a keen eye for human nature. Like Berthold Brecht noticed ninety years ago: 'Food comes first, then morals'." —**Jaap Korteweg**, the Vegetarian Butcher

"Tobias' pragmatism in this book is refreshing. Any method that leads to reduction of used resources, greenhouse gas emissions, and animal suffering should be pursued. Personally, and to illustrate Tobias' points in this book, as a habitual meat-eater, my inclination to become vegetarian or vegan is boosted more by eating in a spectacular vegan restaurant, having a vegetarian daughter, and meeting rational people like Tobias, than my professional endeavors or my encounters with proselytizing vegans."—**Mark Post,** creator of the stemcell-based hamburger

"This book contains many of the ideas I wish I had come by immediately when I went vegan in 2005. It would have saved me and others from countless fruitless discussions. Highly recommended for any vegan who wants to make a difference!"—**Mahi Klosterhalfen**, CEO and president, Albert Schweitzer Foundation

"Through a rational, strategic approach, this book shows the reader how we can all play a part in ending factory farming and sparing billions of animals from suffering."—**David Coman-Hidy,** executive director, The Humane League

"Tobias Leenaert is the meat industry's worst nightmare: a triple-threat visionary who is also utterly pragmatic *and* who writes well. His book is stuffed from beginning to end with great advice that's backed up by research and common sense, and is well delivered. If you care about saving the animals, read it." —**Hillary Rettig**, vegan activist and author, *The Lifelong Activist*

"In a movement charged with emotion, pragmatism can often be overlooked. Tobias takes a critical look at how to create change in our modern society, and his thoughtful viewpoints teach valuable, evidence-based approaches to achieving victories for animals."—**Jon Bockman,** CEO, Animal Charity Evaluators

"I wish *How to Create a Vegan World* fell into my hands years ago. It would have profoundly impacted my views on what helps the most animals. If you care about saving animals you should not only read this book, you should have it on your bedside table."—**Sharon Nuñez**, president, Animal Equality

"*How to Create a Vegan World* is a thoughtful plea for pragmatism in the vegan movement. Drawing on effective altruist principles and social psychology research, Leenaert explores how our biases can blind our advocacy for animals. He makes a powerful case for dropping conventional wisdom and leaving our comfort zone, and instead starting from first principles in our quest to best help animals."—**Lewis Bollard**, farm animal welfare program officer, the Open Philanthropy Project

"People don't do anything when they think they have to do everything. This helpful book provides a practical outline for guiding people to take positive steps and for being the type of activist who asks the question, 'Do I want to be right or do I want to be effective?'"—**Colleen Patrick-Goudreau**, author, *The 30-Day Vegan Challenge*

"Written with precision and clarity, *How to Create a Vegan World* provides sophisticated and unflinching insights that encourage animal advocates to utilize context-driven, unconventional, and often counterintuitive strategies. Tightly-woven layers of thought-provoking ideas champion a broad range of tactics and potential allies intended to sharpen our critical thinking and maximize our impact."—**Dawn Moncrief**, founding director, A Well-Fed World

"*How to Create a Vegan World* delivers some hard truths about our effectiveness as animal advocates. It is thought provocation at its finest. A required read for all pragmatic activists looking for evidenced-based research and strategies that are proven to work."—**Matthew Glover**, cofounder, *Veganuary*

"This book is important in offering a common-sense roadmap to reflect upon as we navigate the complicated path ahead. It is significant in weaving together both theory and research. Tobias' writings have helped shape how I think about my own research and have helped me reconsider how I view veganism and impact."—**Kathryn Asher**, Research Director, Faunalytics; PhD Candidate, University of New Brunswick

How to Create a Vegan World

A Pragmatic Approach

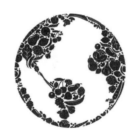

Tobias Leenaert

Illustrations by Amy Hall-Bailey

LANTERN BOOKS • NEW YORK

A Division of Booklight Inc.

2017

Lantern Books
128 Second Place
Brooklyn, NY 11231
www.lanternbooks.com

Printed in the United States of America

Names: Leenaert, Tobias, author.
Title: How to create a vegan world : a pragmatic approach / Tobias Leenaert ; illustrations by Amy Hall-Bailey.
Description: New York : Lantern Books, [2017] | Includes bibliographical references.
Identifiers: LCCN 2017024905 (print) | LCCN 2017019252 (ebook) | ISBN 9781590565711 (ebook) | ISBN 9781590565704 (pbk. : alk. paper)
Subjects: LCSH: Animal welfare—Moral and ethical aspects. | Animal rights. | Veganism.
Classification: LCC HV4708 (print) | LCC HV4708 .L44 2017 (ebook) | DDC 179/.3—dc23

LC record available at https://lccn.loc.gov/2017024905

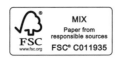

Faith is the bird that feels the light and sings when the dawn is still dark—**Rabindranath Tagore**

CONTENTS

FOREWORD

In the concluding lines of *Animal Liberation*, I wrote:

> Human beings have the power to continue to oppress other species
> forever, or until we make this planet unsuitable for living beings. Will
> our tyranny continue, proving that morality counts for nothing when
> it clashes with self-interest, as the most cynical of poets and philoso-
> phers have always said? Or will we rise to the challenge and prove our
> capacity for genuine altruism by ending our ruthless exploitation of
> the species in our power, not because we are forced to do so by rebels
> or terrorists, but because we recognize that our position is morally
> indefensible?
>
> The answer to this question depends on the way in which each one
> of us, individually, answers it.

More than forty years later, we still don't know the answer to the
question, but the altruists have gained some ground. Across the entire
European Union, from Portugal to Poland and from Finland to Greece,
some of the confinement systems that I described in *Animal Liberation*
have been banned. They have also been banned in California, and major
corporations, like McDonald's and Walmart, have agreed to phase out
their use of products from animals reared by those methods.

Forty years ago, few people even knew what the word *vegan* meant. In
places like Berlin it was difficult to find restaurants that served vegetarian dishes, let alone vegan ones. Now Berlin has a thriving vegan scene,
as do many cities in Europe, North America, Australia, and several other
countries as well. That change has come rapidly, mostly in the past
decade. Vegan food is getting better all the time. Substantial investments
are going into companies that are seeking to grow meat at the cellular
level, or to produce plant-based alternatives that have the same texture
and taste as animal products.

There is, therefore, reason for hope that a major shift toward a vegan world is beginning. In the pages that follow, Tobias Leenaert shows how this hope can be fulfilled. Although the world that he seeks is consistent with the one I was hoping for when I wrote *Animal Liberation*, his approach serves as a useful corrective to the manner in which I posed the question in the lines quoted above. If veganizing the world depends on each one of us choosing altruism over self-interest, then for the foreseeable future the world will be, at best, only partially vegan. I am far from being cynical about the existence of altruism. In working in the animal movement, as well as in the effective altruism movement, I have met people who work incredibly hard in order to reduce the suffering of animals, and I am personally acquainted with three people who have donated their kidneys to complete strangers. But there are also many selfish people in the world, and even more people who, if not exactly selfish, do not extend their ethical gaze beyond themselves, their family, and friends. For these people, the fact that a meal they enjoy causes animals to suffer will not lead them to a different menu choice. Nor will the fact that their meal contributes more to climate change than other meals they could easily choose. They will change only when they are persuaded that it is healthier for them, or more convenient, or less expensive, or perhaps when so many people become vegan that they begin to worry about standing out from the mainstream and being publicly shamed for a diet that has come to seem barbaric.

That is why I now accept that Leenaert is right when he suggests that we are all too prone to believe that there is one correct route to our goal—one road to Veganville, as he calls it—and we know what that route is. There are many routes, and often we don't know which of them will get us to our goal faster. Some of us think we should just tell people about the enormity of our slaughter of animals and the suffering that we inflict on the animals we eat. Once they have that knowledge, surely they have no excuse to avoid turning vegan? Others believe that a gentler, friendlier route will be more successful. They think that we should seek improvements in the welfare of farmed animals, and encourage people to reduce the amount of animal products in their diet. Others, again, prefer not to mention animal suffering, believing that there is a larger audience ready to reduce their carbon footprint. So these advocates argue on the basis of the contribution that animal products make to climate change. Another group thinks that people are more likely to change their behavior if we can persuade them that eating animal products is not good for their health. But, as Leenaert demonstrates, the initial reason why people change is not that important, and the concern for animals may follow later.

We need to test different approaches, and get some reliable data on what works and what doesn't when it comes to persuading people to become vegan. And above all, we need to make it as easy as possible for people to make the change.

There are few people as well-qualified to talk about these issues as Leenaert is. As founder and for ten years director of the Belgian organization Ethical Vegetarian Alternative, he was involved in a campaign that ended with Ghent becoming the first city in the world to officially adopt a weekly "vegetarian day." Then, as codirector (with Melanie Joy) of the Center for Effective Vegan Advocacy, he has run training workshops in vegan advocacy in Europe, South America, South Africa, Asia, and Australia. Now he draws on his wide experience and reading to enable others to become more effective vegan advocates.

One of the things I like best about this book is that Leenaert is under no illusions about the difficulty of reaching his destination of a vegan world, but this does not discourage him from drawing together all the available knowledge about how to get there soonest. If you want to contribute to the vegan movement, and to the better world that it is seeking, this book is an excellent place to start; or if you are already part of that movement, this book will help you to take stock of how well you are doing, and suggest ways in which you can do better. 🌐

Peter Singer
April 2017

INTRODUCTION

The Long Way to Veganville

> "In all affairs it's a healthy thing now and then to hang a question mark on the things you have long taken for granted."
> —attributed to **Bertrand Russell**

To end the killing and suffering of animals at human hands may be one of the greatest challenges ever undertaken by a group of people. If you're reading this book, you are probably part of that group. You might be a vegetarian, a vegan, a meat reducer, or simply a believer or an ally. You might donate to animal causes, or work or volunteer for an animal rights or vegan organization. You could be in business or government, or you might simply want to learn more about how you can help animals. It's my hope that regardless of who you are and what you do, if you want to help create a better world for animals you'll gain new insights from this book.

How to Create a Vegan World presents a pragmatic strategy to guide us toward a tipping point regarding society's attitudes and behavior toward animals, particularly farmed animals. Here's a brief outline of what you'll read.

As I write, all of us are dependent on animals. More and more people around the world eat animal-based meals, sometimes three times a day. I call these people *steakholders*. To change this situation, we cannot mainly or overly rely on persuading them through arguments that appeal to ethics; we'll need to use any means at our disposal. Traditionally, the animal rights (AR) movement has tried to change people's attitudes and motivate them to alter their behavior. The complementary approach I describe in this book is to ask advocates to focus on making behavioral change much easier, so that less motivation is required.

I suggest that we're pragmatic as follows:

- Rather than only using a "Go vegan!" message, we also spend significant resources on encouraging the public to reduce their consumption of animal products. We'll be able to reach the tipping point faster with a mass of reducers than with a small number of vegans.
- We allow people to change for whatever reason they choose, not just because they are persuaded by the moral case for not eating animals. People often change their attitude *after* and not before they alter their behavior.
- We foster an environment that facilitates change, mainly by making the alternatives to animal products better, cheaper, and even more available.
- We develop a more relaxed concept of veganism.

Slow Opinion

We often rush to judgment about issues. The Internet and social media—where it takes only a few seconds to publish a comment or a sneer—contribute to "fast opinion." I'm an enthusiastic proponent of "slow opinion." If you're a "slow opinionist," you're aware of the complexities of life, people, and modern society, and you refuse to form an opinion before you've thought things through and become informed about them.

Slow opinionists don't believe that those on the other side of an argument or issue are necessarily wrong. They won't say *yes* or *no* too fast. Slow opinionists ask questions, and they'll tell the person who currently disagrees with their position that they'll get back to them, after they've taken some time to think about the issue their "opponent" has raised. Slow opinion is also about empathy. It's about wondering what it's like to be in the other person's shoes. Slow opinionists ask themselves about other people: *What values are important for them? What positions are they in? Could they perhaps have a good reason to say, write, or do this?* One of the greatest advantages of slow opinion is it can reduce judgmentalism and blanket condemnation of other people (including those we love to hate, such as politicians and celebrities) and their opinions.

The animal advocacy and vegan movements could benefit a lot from slow opinion and deep thinking. We could stand to be less judgmental—of people on our side as well as those on the other. Slow opinion would help us to refine our strategies to influence people positively.

For many of my fellow animal advocates and vegans, the approach I set out in this book will appear to break the rules and diverge from well-trodden paths. But I believe that everything—even our most heartfelt beliefs—should be scrutinized on occasion, so we can make sure we're on the right track and continuously improve our tactics and strategies. Even if you may not agree with everything you read, I suggest you keep an open mind, and be a slow opinionist.

FINDING OUT WHAT WORKS

Slow opinion may make us more deliberative and strategic, but I don't want our openness to nuance and uncertainty to paralyze us. That's why we need to conduct due diligence in finding out what works. Sometimes we may need to test approaches we're not sure of, to see if they move us closer to our goal or not.

In Steven Spielberg's movie *Lincoln*, the eponymous hero and Representative Thaddeus Stevens discuss how to pass the amendment that will abolish slavery. Stevens talks about our "inner compass" and how it should point North, showing us where to go and what is right. Regrettably, he adds, many people's compass is off. This is Lincoln's reply:

> A compass, I learned when I was surveying, it'll . . . it'll point you True North from where you're standing, but it's got no advice about the swamps and deserts and chasms that you'll encounter along the way. If in pursuit of your destination, you plunge ahead, heedless of obstacles, and achieve nothing more than to sink in a swamp . . . what's the use of knowing True North? (Tuttle)

Lincoln (at least in the film) is wily and shrewd, although his caution and deliberation infuriate those who feel the moral imperatives of their cause demand direct action. Lincoln knows that effective strategies or tactics are those that help us get to our goal as fast as possible; they may not necessarily be the straightest or purest, or, for that matter, the most obvious.

When discussing strategies, many of us are likely to commit one of two errors. The first is to believe that there's *one* correct approach. People and society are obviously too varied and complicated for that to be true. The second is the opposite of the first: it's to think that *all* strategies are useful and necessary. Some will work better than others, and we want to invest our limited resources in the best or most promising of them. We shouldn't be satisfied with true but trivial statements like "different approaches will work for different people." If we only persuade one person when we could have persuaded a thousand, we've wasted our efforts, unless of course that one person carries considerable influence in society. Moreover, it's possible that some strategies could do more harm than good. If a strategy appeals to one hundred people but alienates a thousand others, it's probably not effective.

If we want to know which strategies, tactics, or campaigns are more successful than others, we cannot simply rely on our personal experiences, gut feelings, or intuition. They have their place, but we need to support them with data from proven research. Our assumptions about what drives or affects other people are often wrong, and we are prone to many biases.

In sum, we need to think things through. We should conduct research and collect data and evidence even if we can't expect definitive outcomes or answers to *all* our questions. We should take into account many different factors, parameters, and unknowns across a wide range of types of research. Some researchers, whether from organizations or academic institutions, may measure people's reactions to statements and images, their psychological predispositions and motivations, how they "click" online, and other behaviors. Some may study the history of other social movements for lessons valuable to our own. We can also use results from studies of other topics, like psychology or social science, or even marketing, innovation, and other disciplines. The insights we gather through all these methods help us improve our efforts to create the changes we want.

For this book, I've relied as much as possible on research featured in the previous paragraph, and have referenced my statements as such. Most of what I present is backed up by evidence of various degrees of strength. The rest is more speculative, and may or may not be confirmed by future research. Part of the function of this book is to raise questions to stimulate your thinking and to encourage further research.

EFFECTIVE ALTRUISM

Effective altruism (EA) is a philosophy and movement whose proponents apply scientific research and evidence to reduce suffering and increase happiness. The EA movement is not only playing a major role in further mainstreaming the issue of cruelty to animals, but it's had a significant influence on animal advocacy itself in the last few years. EA concepts and ideas have helped the AR movement focus more on effectiveness by emphasizing the different criteria we should take into account when we make choices and assess our influence. Such criteria are the amount and the intensity of suffering, the resources that are already invested in a certain problem (is it, in other words, neglected?), and whether there are good and clear solutions to that problem.

One EA organization within the domain of animal advocacy is Animal Charity Evaluators, which seeks to discover and advocate for effective methods to improve the lives of animals. Also instrumental in making animal advocacy more evidence-based and results-oriented are books by Nick Cooney (*Veganomics, Change of Heart, How to Be Great at Doing Good*) and the organization Faunalytics. See the Appendix and Bibliography for more details. ∎

The Road to Veganville

Throughout this book, I use a metaphor to illustrate my argument and clarify different concepts. It makes the strategy easier to remember.

Veganville is an imaginary town on top of a mountain. Most of you reading this book may live there already. But, if you do, your (and my) aim is to get as many other people as we can to live with us, as soon as possible. Like all metaphors, this one isn't perfect—for one thing, our town would be extremely crowded—but it serves a purpose. Below, the different parts of the metaphor are explained in more detail.

- In chapter 1, *Getting Our Bearings*, we take a look at where we want to go and where exactly we are at the moment. From a brief look at the present situation, I conclude that our movement needs a high dose of pragmatism. In each of the next chapters I explain how to be pragmatic.

- In chapter 2, *The Call to Action*, we examine what we should ideally ask people in order to get them to start moving. It might appear that the most obvious thing to tell them would be, "Come to us. Right now!" But, following Lincoln's logic, perhaps there are different roads to Veganville, or we can tell people to make the journey in stages; or they can visit on daytrips.

- Chapter 3, *Arguments*, asks which reasons we can or should use to encourage others to join us. People need to hike for many days uphill to arrive at Veganville. We know it's worth the effort, but they don't—at least not yet. How best to motivate them?

- Chapter 4, *Environment*, is about everything external to our travelers. We'll need to improve the roads, and make sure that there are lodges, resting places, and assistants should they need some help en route.

- Chapter 5, *Support*, is about us coming down from the mountain and encouraging people to start and keep climbing. It's about our day-to-day interactions and communication with them. In this chapter I also take a closer look at how we should define veganism.

- Chapter 6, *Sustainability,* is about ensuring that once our travelers have made it, they stay, and that those who help others climb the mountain don't burn out.

(In the illustration of the road to Veganville below [Fig. 1], the numbers indicate the chapters in the book.)

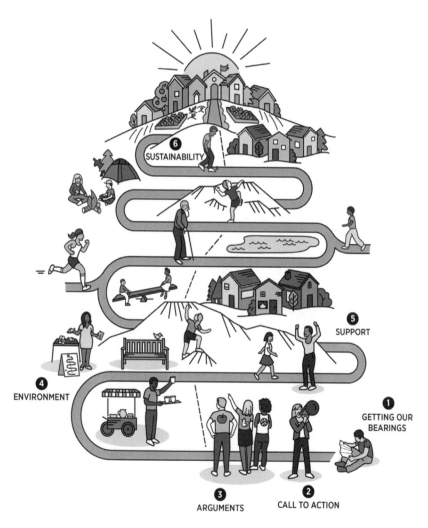

Fig. 1: The Road to Veganville

On Terms and Scope

Though animals suffer and are killed for more than just our eating habits, I mainly focus on decreasing the consumption and production of animal foods. Animal agriculture is the most far-reaching and consequential form of animal exploitation. It accounts for 99 percent of the animals killed by humans, and many more animals die in the food industry than through scientific research, hunting, or the clothing and entertainment industries combined.

When I talk about *meat*, I'm usually referring to *meat and other animal products*, including fish, dairy, and eggs, just as *meat reducers* stands for *reducers of animal products*. When I write about *vegans*, I also include vegetarians. When the difference between both is significant, I write *vegetarians and vegans*. With *the vegan movement* or *the animal rights movement* I describe a diverse and ever-shifting group of people that wishes to minimize animal killing, suffering, and injustice (we'll talk about the exact aim in the next several pages), even though they may differ slightly about the end goal, and much more about how to get there. I don't want to exclude people who are specifically or mainly motivated by concerns for their health from carrying the VEGAN label. Indeed, I don't believe that's strategic. For the purpose of this book, however, when I talk about *the vegan movement* I'm thinking of those who are motivated by a belief that it is unethical to utilize animals for food, clothing, and other purposes. I include myself among them—with some caveats, as you will read.

My examples mainly come from the movement in Europe and North America. Most available research is conducted from these regions, especially the US. Sometimes, facts and data can be extrapolated to other regions; sometimes they can't or shouldn't. (In North America and Europe, consumption of animal products is stagnating or declining; in developing countries it is often rising, fast.)

Finally, for brevity's sake, I use the term *animals* rather than *nonhuman animals*. ☺

1

Getting Our Bearings

Where Are We Going, and Where Are We?

"Speed is irrelevant if you're going in the wrong direction."
—**Mohandas K. Gandhi**

If we want everyone to move to Veganville, we need to have an idea of the situation we're in right now. How many people live down the mountain? What are they thinking and feeling? Is it easy for them to start the journey? What is the condition of the roads? Translated to the vegan movement, these questions involve public support for our goal, the ideas people have about animals, how available alternatives are, the obstacles to going vegan, and what motivates vegans. Before looking at the present situation though, let's briefly examine how much we agree on our ultimate goals, because these are not as obvious as they may appear.

The Goals of This Movement

In the most general terms, we in the vegan movement want to *help* as many animals as much as possible. What in this context does *helping* mean? Here are three ways to address that issue. Helping could mean:

(1) Reducing as much animal suffering as possible
(2) Reducing as much killing as possible
(3) Reducing injustice toward animals as much as possible

I will assume that most readers of this book will agree with numbers one and two. I'm aware that many people consider it acceptable to kill animals if it's performed painlessly and the animal had "a good life" (whatever that means), but the audience I keep in mind for this book are the people who find slaughtering animals for food, clothing, or pleasure to be objectionable and want to abolish it.

The third number on our list is trickier. Some of our actions toward, or relationships with, animals that could be considered speciesist[1] or that infringe on animals' alleged rights, aren't necessarily harmful. There can be, for instance, discussion about horseback-riding, backyard egg-laying hens, or even companion animals, such as dogs and cats. Personally, I'm against almost all use of animals, mainly because I want to protect them from suffering and/or being killed. Animals may not be entirely free, but that doesn't necessarily mean they're being harmed (not all "use" constitutes "abuse"). Conversely, animals living freely in nature may at times be subjected to extreme suffering (see box on p. 11).

It's beyond the scope of this book to engage in a lengthy philosophical discussion about the ultimate aims of the animal advocacy movement, beyond the three goals listed above. I take it as a given that vegans and animal advocates to a large extent would agree with these goals and want to bring their realization closer.

A vegan world, therefore, is one where animals aren't made to suffer or killed wantonly by humans, and where almost all use of animals has been abolished, although some mutually beneficial relationships between humans and animals may remain. By this definition, a vegan world is not the goal in itself, just as veganism is not an end in itself, but a vehicle for that vision.

A Double Demand

If we in the vegan movement examine what we ask of nonvegans, we'll notice that we desire two different things. First, we want others to change their *behavior*: to stop consuming animal products. Secondly, we also want them to alter their *attitude*: to stop consuming animal products *because they care about animals*. In other words, we don't just want people to do the right thing; we want them to do the right thing *for the right reasons*. To clarify even further: Imagine a world in which no one ate animal products since they've become redundant as "resources," and

Wild Animal Suffering

Animals in the wild experience starvation, predation, disease, parasites, and adverse climatic conditions—independently of human action or inaction. This reality usefully illustrates the differences between focusing on suffering (and killing) on the one hand, and justice, fairness, autonomy, and other values on the other. Even if we focus on abolishing injustice, all of these natural realities will remain.

The difficult truth for many of us to swallow is that the *cause* of suffering—human or not—is irrelevant for those experiencing it. It makes no difference to a rabbit whether she suffers because of some terrible disease, or because she was caught in a trap set by a human being. The disease might actually entail more suffering, but it is only the trapper, and not nature or predators, who can be guilty of committing a moral infraction. The point of this story is that seeing suffering as the bottom line may lead us to interfere (when possible and effective) in nature. The values we focus on can make a difference in our actions and advocacy. ■

more available, cheaper, healthier alternatives are available. I'm fairly sure that most vegan activists, like myself, might not feel entirely comfortable in this "accidentally vegan" world. We'd want people to be motivated by a moral concern, not just because such attitudes appear to be the basis for permanent change, but also because being moral is valuable in itself. We want an "intentionally vegan" world, where people hold ethical values and attitudes about animals as possessing inherent and non-instrumental rights; where, indeed, they give up the habits and traditions that appear to drive so much of our meat consumption and become conscious about their food choices.

The illustration on the next page (Fig. 2) shows what most of us in the movement want: for people to go vegan because they like animals. All other options—even being vegan for other reasons—appear to us less than ideal (hence the unhappy faces).

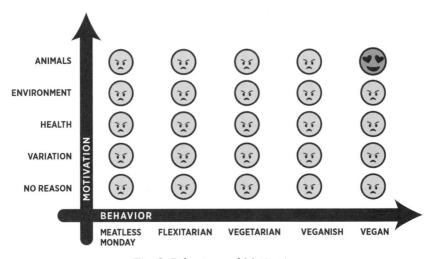

Fig. 2: Behavior and Motivation

Both behavior and attitudes are important. However, as I explain in the following chapters, we don't need to ask for both at the same time and we don't need this double demand in all our messages.

Now that we have an idea of where we want to go, let's take a look at the situation today.

Too Many "Steakholders"

The enormous amount of animal product consumed is enabled, supported, and perpetuated by a massive, economically significant industry. To get an idea of the economic value generated by animals solely in the area of food products, we must take into account primary production (people earning their money by raising pigs, cows, chickens, and other animals); growers of animal feed; companies that manufacture farm equipment; the pharmaceutical industry, which sells antibiotics and other drugs to growers; veterinarians and food inspectors; slaughterhouses; transportation; supermarkets; and restaurants and caterers, among others.

In his book *Changing the Game*, the late Norm Phelps, after some number crunching, and combining farming, post-farming processing, and retail sales, arrives at a direct yearly revenue of $2.74 trillion in the

United States alone. Compare this to the "mere" $734 billion in direct annual revenues in the automotive industry—including manufacturing, sales, and service (p. 45). We can add to this number a whole culture of chefs, cookbook writers, food-preparation contests, culinary lessons, and many other sectors or subsectors that rely on animal products for at least a part of their turnover or success. And we haven't even started to mention animals in clothing, entertainment, or research.

This sketch makes clear how dependent our society is on the use of animals. One could almost say that this planet, or humanity, is "powered by animals." To my knowledge, no study has been carried out on the degree of dependence, but it would seem to dwarf our exploitation of the free labor of enslaved people, women, or children. This dependency is fundamental and needs to be tackled. Yet it's not easy to change something if you are, or think you are, wholly dependent on it. In fact, it's not too far-fetched to say that, at this point in time, animal (ab)use may be too substantial a part of our culture and economy for it to be abandoned, even if the whole world agreed with us that the present state of affairs was problematic.

That systemic reality may well contribute to the reason why, for most individuals, accepting that a shift away from animals is necessary and implementing that awareness in practice is so hard. Further reasons are covered by psychologist Melanie Joy's "three N's of justification" (Joy 2010; Piazza et al. 2015):

- *Eating animals is normal.* Animal products are on almost all menus, in all supermarkets, in cooking shows on TV, and in many other areas of everyday life.
- *Eating animals is natural.* We have been eating meat and using animals for tens of thousands of years, and just like many animals kill and eat other animals, to most people it only seems natural that *Homo sapiens* also kills and eats other species.
- *Eating animals is necessary.* Whereas many people may consider it sad that we raise and kill animals for food, they are convinced that we need to eat meat, or at least some animal products, in

order to thrive. Concern for one's health is one of the main factors that keep people from going or staying vegetarian or vegan, while at the same time health is a big motivator for many people to reduce their intake of animal products (Faunalytics 2012; Cooney 2014, p. 81; Piazza et al. 2015).

A fourth "N" to consider is that many people find eating animal products *nice*, or delicious. Next to health concerns, taste is the other main reason why people don't go vegetarian (Faunalytics 2012; Cooney 2014, p. 82; Mullee et al. 2017). They don't want to miss out on their juicy steak, and find the alternatives—insofar as they've tried them—unsatisfying. If animal products are natural, normal, necessary, and nice, a shift away from animal products—let alone giving them up entirely—seems unnatural, abnormal, unnecessary, and unattractive.

CREATURES OF CONFORMITY

In the 1950s, the American psychologist Solomon E. Asch recruited participants at Swarthmore College in Pennsylvania for a now-famous experiment (Asch 1951, 1956). Asch told his study subjects that he was researching perception. In reality, he was conducting a study about conformity and social pressure.

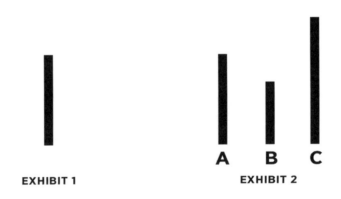

EXHIBIT 1   **EXHIBIT 2**

Fig. 3: Solomon Asch's Conformity Experiment

Asch showed the participants a set of pictures like the one in Fig. 3. He then asked them which of the three bars on the right was the same length as the one on the left. (It's not an optical illusion: the correct answer is obviously A.) Participants had to answer out loud in the group, one by one. However, all but one of the group members were conspirators, whom Asch had ordered to provide the same, incorrect answer. The sole real, unsuspecting participant had to answer after all the others. To his surprise, Asch found that in this situation over a third (37 percent) of respondents provided an incorrect answer, compared to just one percent in the control group. When asked to explain why, some people said they thought the group was correct. Other respondents were afraid of appearing different or didn't want to cause any trouble. Asch concluded: "The tendency to conformity in our society is so strong that reasonably intelligent and well-meaning young people are willing to call white black" (Asch 1955, p. 5).

It's not difficult to transfer these findings to our own domain. Research shows that 63 percent of former vegetarians and vegans disliked that their diet made them stick out from the crowd (Asher et al. 2014). Even aside from the need to conform, it's evident that when a large majority of people think differently from you, it's hard for anyone to be entirely convinced of his or her own dissident thoughts. When people constantly see that consuming animal products is considered normal, it's tough for them even to believe in the vague discomfort that they may be experiencing, and it becomes a lot more difficult to think that something wrong is occurring. Even if you're already a vegetarian or vegan, and you've internalized the principle that it's problematic to eat animal products, you may have these moments of doubt, wondering if you're actually seeing things correctly. South African–born author and Nobel Laureate J. M. Coetzee attributes the following thoughts to his vegetarian character Elizabeth Costello:

> It's that I no longer know where I am. I seem to move around perfectly easily among people, to have perfectly normal relations with them. Is it possible, I ask myself, that all of them are participants in a crime of

stupefying proportions? Am I fantasizing it all? I must be mad! Yet every day I see the evidences. The very people I suspect produce the evidence, exhibit it, offer it to me. Corpses. Fragments of corpses that they have bought for money. . . . Yet I'm not dreaming. I look into your eyes . . . and I see only kindness, human kindness. Calm down, I tell myself, you are making a mountain out of a molehill. This is life. Everyone else comes to terms with it, why can't you? *Why can't you?* (Coetzee)

In part because only a tiny minority of people consider meat eating problematic or act differently, most people don't consciously stop to think about meat eating as a moral issue, let alone behave accordingly. Psychologist Steven Pinker considers it one of the major conclusions of social psychology that "people take their cues on how to behave from other people" (p. 674). To the question of why most people eat meat, one answer that we can give is the following:

> ## MOST PEOPLE EAT MEAT
> ### because
> ## MOST PEOPLE EAT MEAT.

Even if one came to the conclusion that eating animals is wrong, turning the realization into practice is not easy. People are afraid they will stand out too much, or be inconvenienced, or suffer from poor health, or there will be nothing tasty left to eat—to name a few fears and concerns. All in all, it appears that the great majority of people have no intention of eliminating meat, much less other animal products (Faunalytics 2007, Ivox), and that even if they do consider it, many believe it difficult to accomplish. As Matt Ball writes: "No one sits around thinking, 'Wow, I really want to give up all my favorite foods and be different from my friends and family!'" (2014, p. 112) Going vegan still means an uphill struggle—which is why in our metaphor Veganville is situated on top of a mountain.

Vegans who disagree and say that going vegan *is* easy are probably looking at things only from their viewpoint. We'll talk later about putting ourselves in others' shoes. For now, if you don't believe going vegan is hard for many, consider that, according to research by Faunalytics, even *staying* vegan is hard: 84 percent of vegetarians or vegans at some point abandon their diet (Asher et al. 2014). I return to this in chapter 6.

Our Cause Is Different

Strategic activists "are aware of and sensitive to the uniqueness of the movement," writes Melanie Joy in *Strategic Action for Animals*. One central consideration for vegan advocates is to remember that our struggle is notably different from any other prior effort. Vegans like to compare our struggle to human rights causes, past and present: such as the campaign to end slavery, women's liberation, the fight against racism, and gay rights. Certainly, there are similarities, and animal liberation can be considered a social justice movement like these, where we attempt to raise the status of the oppressed so they can receive equal consideration of their interests under the law (Nibert).

Furthermore, parallels can be drawn between how ideological belief systems, such as racism and sexism, justify prejudices toward human "out-groups" on the one hand and how we treat and think about animals on the other (Regan, Singer 1995, Spiegel; Joy 2010). People who see a greater difference between humans and animals (Costello and Hodson 2010, 2014) or endorse more speciesist attitudes (Dhont et al.) at the same time show more prejudice toward immigrant or ethnic out-groups. Our understanding of human intergroup relations may help us to understand human–animal relations (Dhont and Hodson 2015).

Still, although comparisons with other movements offer useful means whereby people can see or think about animals differently, we shouldn't lose sight of the distinctions or automatically assume we can transplant lessons from other movements to our own. Below, I take a quick look at some of the unique challenges of animal advocacy.

ANIMALS ARE NOT PEOPLE

Whether *we* see relevant differences between nonhuman and human animals or not, most of our fellow human beings do. Anti-speciesist arguments are often elegant, powerful, and sensible, but as yet, most people aren't buying them. All other movements—except for some aspects of environmentalism, which are in any event often anthropocentric—are about people. It's true that women, people of color, or non-heterosexuals have been or sometimes are still considered out-groups, and that members of certain of these out-groups at some periods and places in history weren't even considered human at all. Yet it's easier to see similarities between different kinds of people than between people and animals. Animals are perhaps the original out-group, the ultimate "other."

In spite of the similarities between power dynamics among human groups and between humans and animals, most people don't consider this connection relevant (Costello and Hodson 2014). Some studies show that comparing humans to animals may be ineffective in improving people's attitudes toward animals (Costello and Hodson 2010). People with traditional cultural values in particular may view veganism as a threat to their social status and the norms of mainstream culture. It's possible that animal rights advocacy could actually foster more speciesism and meat consumption as an active "push-back" against the growing success of the vegan movement (Dhont and Hodson 2014, 2015).

FIGHTING WITHOUT THE VICTIMS

"We are attempting to be the first social justice movement in history to succeed without the organized, conscious participation of the victims," writes Norm Phelps (p. 25). The number of humans campaigning for animals is still small: more than 95 percent of the population isn't yet onboard with the minority's vision, let alone practice. A lot more support will be required to change the system, and it's not going to come from the animals, who'll never revolt like they do in George Orwell's *Animal Farm* or in the animated movie *Chicken Run*.

To be clear, in every movement the privileged have fought for or along-side the oppressed—sometimes in leading roles, sometimes as support-ers. Yet at the least, a critical mass of the oppressed was involved in the fight. To make matters worse, the fact that we speak for others poses a challenge in itself. Melanie Joy writes: "Direct victims have much more moral authority to call attention to their own suffering; they are often allowed and even expected to be outraged and outspoken. On the other hand, advocates of victims appear moralistic when they speak out on behalf of the victims" (2008, p. 45).

CHANGING SOMETHING ANCIENT

Our attitudes around food are notoriously difficult to change. Most readers will know how hard it is to say *no* to food we know isn't good for us, or to avoid eating too much of it. (That third or fourth vegan donut *still* looks tasty!) Reducing people's meat consumption may be even tougher. In her book *Meathooked*, journalist Marta Zaraska goes on a quest to explain why so many of us are addicted to meat. She writes about the role meat may have played in our evolution, and how the sharing of it helped build communities. Whether we like it or not, meat has for millennia been special to us, in addition to being a convenient means of bringing us valuable protein. Zaraska also searches for the compounds in meat that make it so attractive and sometimes addictive to people. (Spoiler alert: it's the fat, the aromas, and the umami taste.) She explains how the origins of what we like to eat can be sourced from our time in the womb, when we develop a liking for what our mother eats, and later for what comes through our mother's milk.

Most people are aware that their diet affects their health, other people, animals, and our planet. But growing up routinely eating animal products and liking the taste and convenience, these individuals rarely consider the consequences and/or animal-free foods as an alternative. Plant-based foods are seen by many as lacking in taste, range, and availability. The pro-vegan organization ProVeg International, of which I am a cofounder (see box "Influencing the Influencers" on p. 98), calls this phenomenon "veg prejudice." Veg prejudice keeps many people from translating their knowledge into actions.

Meat also has symbolic value. In *Some We Love, Some We Hate, Some We Eat*, professor of psychology and anthrozoology Hal Herzog quotes the owner of a barbecue restaurant as follows: "It's been ingrained in our heads that sitting down and eating a good piece of meat is a sign of success. It makes your mind feel good" (p. 180). Whether what the man is saying is scientifically grounded or not, his sentiment is probably close to how many people, on some level, feel about eating meat. Especially men. As many authors have demonstrated, meat stands for virility, and not eating it isn't considered manly (see Zaraska, Fiddes, Adams). Then, there is the role meat plays in our culture and the place it occupies at our social gatherings. To a degree, the animal-products industry has an easy task. They are telling us, offering us, seducing us with what most of us want to hear—animal foods are desirable, normal, healthy, and tasty.

A Time for Pragmatism

"Pragmatism asks its usual question. 'Grant an idea or belief to be true,' it says, 'what concrete difference will its being true make in anyone's actual life? How will the truth be realized? What experiences will be different from those which would obtain if the belief were false? What, in short, is the truth's cash-value?'"—**William James**

It should be clear by now that weaning society off meat is a massive task. As individuals and a society we're incredibly invested in and dependent on using animals. This truth—combined with the unique challenges of vegan animal advocacy—makes change slow and difficult. Even though we're growing and professionalizing our organizations, vegetarians and vegans occupy no more than a couple of percent of the adult population in even the most "advanced" countries in this respect. Although our experience might feel different, the number of vegans hasn't risen spectacularly in

I Was Meathooked

I remember thinking I should stop eating meat because I loved animals when I was eight or ten years old. I looked at my dog lying cozily near the fireplace while a cow grazed in the rain outside, destined for slaughter. I wondered why I petted one and ate the other. I couldn't find any morally relevant factor to explain this different treatment of these two species and concluded that logically I should stop eating animals. Still, I didn't change, because I loved the taste of meat and it was too inconvenient to stop eating it. Attempts by my health-conscious mother to take me to vegetarian restaurants, as well as her cooking vegetarian meals now and then, met with a lot of resistance on my part. My first choice when eating out was invariably *steak au poivre*.

Whenever I was confronted with a vegetarian (I didn't know any vegans at the time), all my defense mechanisms sprang into action. I didn't want to know. I didn't want to change. Yet I couldn't deny that what I was doing was not what I wanted for the animals. During my college years, I read Peter Singer's *Animal Liberation* and became even more conflicted. A non-vegetarian friend who knew about my uneasiness at eating meat made me a bet: if I went a month without eating meat or fish, he'd give me what amounted to $25—otherwise I'd have to pay that amount to him. I won the bet without much difficulty. Afterward, I *still* didn't become entirely vegetarian: I decided to eat no meat, except for that in pasta dishes, which, as a student, were an inevitable staple. I also still ate fish. Then I stopped eating meat in pasta, and later the fish. Two years later (now almost two decades ago) I became a vegan.

So I know what it's like. Even when you *want* to change your diet, when you're sitting down with a menu in front of you, it's easy to say: *Not this time. This time, I will just pick what I know I will enjoy. Change is for tomorrow.* ∎

the last few decades (VRG). Hal Herzog's assessment is not one we can be cheerful about: "In spite of what you sometimes hear, over the past thirty years, the animal rights movement has not made much of a dent in our desire to dine on other species" (p. 176). Veganville seems to be impossibly far away for most people, on a mountain too high to climb. Meanwhile, our opponents are trying to prevent people starting the trek, investing literally billions of dollars in advertising to keep them hooked on meat.[2]

In the present context, therefore, focusing only on trying to make people go vegan for animals or to tell them to become anti-speciesists won't be enough. Norm Phelps, writing in 2014, says:

> This is not a time when we can expect direct strategies to bring success. This is a time for indirect strategies; for planting seeds that will bear fruit in the future. . . . This is a time for gathering strength and laying the groundwork for future success. (p. 64)

It is, in short, a time to be highly pragmatic. Pragmatism, according to the Cambridge Essential English Dictionary, is the quality of dealing with a problem in a manner that suits the conditions that really exist, rather than following fixed theories, ideas, or rules. Being pragmatic, then, is about reality rather than rules. Finding a good word for the opposite of pragmatism is difficult. *Dogmatism* has too negative a connotation, while another candidate, *idealism*, seems overly positive. I suggest we consider a spectrum like this (Fig. 4):

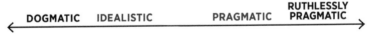

Fig. 4: The Spectrum from Idealism to Pragmatism

Moving too far along the spectrum in either direction can be problematic. Dogma is dangerous and unproductive, but if you go too far in the other direction you risk compromising too much or being unethical in achieving your goals. I will use the word *idealistic* as the opposite of *pragmatic*, keeping in mind that dogmatism may always be just around the corner.

Let me illustrate the difference between pragmatism and idealism with the example of the Meatless (or Meatfree) Monday campaign. I write more on this later, but for now let's assume there are good reasons to believe this campaign can bring us closer to our goal. Those with a pragmatic attitude would then be in favor of it, as they are most concerned with the question, *Does this work?* Those on the other side of the spectrum, however, may have problems with asking people to go meatfree for one day a week. If we believe that killing animals is morally wrong, so the reasoning goes, we can't implicitly condone it by implying that it's OK to eat animals the other six days of the week. (The same argument could be made in terms of vegan versus vegetarian. Meatless doesn't mean vegan.) This doesn't conform to the idealists' belief. They'll say asking for Meatless Mondays isn't right, and therefore shouldn't be advocated for.

Now, although these different positions may lead to two different outcomes, such as supporting the Meatless Monday campaign or not, it's important to note that the idealists—who are focused on "rightness"—don't necessarily ignore effectiveness. Indeed, they may think that the campaign doesn't work. What's more, idealists often believe that doing what's morally right will lead to the best result, or conversely, that something that is not right in their eyes cannot work. But this is fantasy rather than fact. Similarly, pragmatists—who are focused on "effectiveness"—agree with the principle of not using animals and don't ignore "rightness." So we can see that both pragmatists and idealists find both effectiveness and rightness (the results and the principles) valuable. It's only their focus that's different. No one is purely focused on results, and no one is purely focused on rules or principles. Everyone but the most ruthless pragmatist has principles that they'll never break. All but the most dogmatic idealist will agree that in certain situations we may need to prioritize impact and temporarily suspend a principle. (See page 40 for further discussion of Meatless Mondays.)

The table below gives you a possible further description of both an idealistic and pragmatic approach in the vegan movement. Keep in mind that we're talking about a spectrum rather than a strict dichotomy.

	IDEALISTIC	PRAGMATIC
Ultimate goal	Ending animal killing/suffering/injustice	
Strategic goal	More vegans	Reduction of consumption
Call to action	A call to action that confirms the end goal: "Go vegan"	A call to action that can contribute to the goal: "reduce," "eat more plant-based," "do Meatless Monday," "go vegetarian"
Arguments	For the animals	For any reason (animals, health, taste, sustainability)
Focus	Focus on personal values, duties, morals	Focus also on the alternatives/surroundings
Partners	Exclusive: collaborate with like-minded people	Inclusive: collaborate with anyone who can make a contribution to the goal
Welfare reforms	Welfare reforms not advocated or even supported	(Most) welfare reforms welcome or at least not opposed

It's unfortunately quite typical for social movements to become polarized. The more idealistic camp takes a position against the more pragmatic, and vice versa. Idealists may tell pragmatists they're sell-outs, that they're resorting to means that aren't justified by the ends, or that they're deviating more and more from the objective. Erik Marcus on his website vegan.com writes that "one of the costs of being a pragmatist is that others are always questioning your integrity and your motivation."

Some Thought Experiments: Idealistic or Pragmatic?

You can test to what extent you take a more idealistic or pragmatic approach by asking yourself what you'd do in the situations below.

Eating at nonvegan restaurants. From an idealistic viewpoint, you may want to avoid spending any money on businesses that aren't vegan (if you have the choice). These businesses might invest your money in more products that entail animal suffering. From a more pragmatic viewpoint, you could reason that if business owners notice that there's a demand for vegan products or meals, they might increase their number and variety, so that many other customers might try the vegan products rather than the animal ones. This question can also apply to larger economic choices. Imagine that a mainly omnivorous fast-food chain tests a new vegan burger. As an activist in a vegan organization, knowing that your group can make a major difference, do you suggest to your members and followers that they purchase the burger to boost sales so it rolls out nationally, thus allowing many meat eaters to choose it instead of their usual meat burger?

The great vegetarian burger and the awful vegan burger. Envisage a situation in which you can buy lunch for a really hungry nonvegan friend, whom we'll call Bill. The restaurant offers two meatless choices: a great-tasting vegetarian burger (it has some egg in it to bind it), and a terrible-tasting vegan burger. Which one do you pick? From an idealistic viewpoint, you may reason that you cannot allow yourself to buy or even recommend anything nonvegan. Pragmatically, you may decide that if Bill eats the bad vegan burger, he may undergo an experience that will literally and metaphorically leave a negative taste in his mouth. This may make Bill less likely to become more open to trying other vegan products and to lose his "veg prejudice" in the future. Eating a tasty vegetarian burger, on the other hand, would mean some complicity in animal suffering, but the psychological effect of a person thinking *Is that meatfree? That's yummy!* is probably much more catalytic and valuable in the long run. ∎

Pragmatists, for their part, may tell idealists they've gotten mired in their own set of rules and have lost touch with the real world, which makes them ineffective. In the worst case, people on different ends of the spectrum will actively oppose one another.

When I argue that this is a time for considerable pragmatism, I mean a time will come when a more idealistic approach is appropriate. How pragmatic or idealistic a movement can or should be depends to a large extent on what phase it's in. Over time, as public support for our cause grows and dependence on the use of animals decreases, the importance of pragmatism will diminish, and idealistic messages will become more productive and necessary. We can present this as follows (Fig. 5):

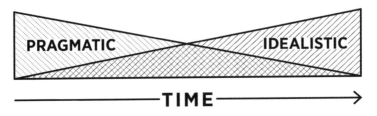

Fig. 5: Pragmatism and Idealism over Time

One Vegan's Activist Trajectory

In the course of your life as an advocate, you may change your approach and your beliefs about what is appropriate or effective. Let me describe the phases I myself have gone through in almost twenty years of activism.

1. Interest and Conversion

After a long period lurking at the back of my mind, "going veg" finally came to the fore. My principal reason was the cruel treatment of animals. (Others might be concerned with their health, or worried about the effects of animal agriculture on the environment, or because their significant other is vegan.) I began to leave animal products out of my diet. After two years, from 1998 onward, I started calling myself a vegan.

2. ACTIVATION

I continued to read about the horrors of animal abuse and decided I needed to do something more. I became passionate about the cause and wanted to help the world become vegan. By now, I fully believed in animal liberation. I wrote my master's degree thesis about it, and took up internships in four different animal rights organizations in the United States immediately after graduation.

3. RADICALIZATION

After a while I grew frustrated and occasionally angry at people's unresponsiveness in the face of so much injustice and suffering. I got to know different people in the vegan movement and read articles and books that presented a starkly black-and-white view of veganism. I decided there was "no excuse for animal abuse" and that people should become vegans as soon as they knew the facts. I criticized some animal rights organizations who take a pragmatic position, and considered them sell-outs, "welfarist,"[3] and too soft. I questioned their motives.

4. REALIZATION

After more reading, thinking, and meeting people, I *realized* the approach I was taking wasn't the most effective, and became more *realistic* and pragmatic, without changing or betraying any of my principles. I concluded that people needed more than just moral persuasion, and that encouragement works better than guilt-tripping. I noticed, and kept noticing, how many people around me changed their eating habits without me preaching to them. I also realized that most people working for animal rights organizations are well-intentioned and are doing important work. ■

CONCLUSION

The question of what works and what doesn't always needs to be answered in the light of circumstances: What is happening where you are and when? Any strategy that works well today may not in ten years' time. Conversely, some strategies or campaigns may not be ideal today, but may become useful in the future—when there is, it might be hoped, more public support for more radical action.

Because of humans' extreme dependency on using animals, the uniqueness of the animal advocates' challenge, the fact that we're relatively few in number, and the great opposition to our cause, vegans need a high dose of pragmatism. Within that context, I suggest in the following chapters that:

- We are pragmatic in what we ask of people
- We are pragmatic in the reasons we give people to change
- We create an environment that facilitates change
- We apply a more relaxed concept of veganism

It's easy to be a philosopher and say true things about the rights of animals. It's much harder to get your hands dirty and do the right things at the right time truly to make a difference. That's the art of high-impact advocacy. ✪

2

THE CALL TO ACTION

What Do We Ask People to Do?

"One may walk over the highest mountain one step at a time."
—**John Wanamaker**

We agree that we want as many people as possible to come to live in Veganville. But does it follow from this desire that "Join us in Veganville!" is *the* message we should deliver? What if we can suggest something that sounds more attractive and more achievable? What if we provided some in-between goals? Or maybe we can tell visitors they don't have to reach Veganville but that living anywhere on the mountain will be wonderful. They'd have a terrific view and receive many of the benefits of living near Veganville! Or what if we ask people just to visit us? Rather than buying or building a house in Veganville, we can offer them a month at a hotel or resort, and see how they like it.

In a time when people in more and more countries are entirely meathooked, what should we ideally ask them to do? Go vegan? Go vegetarian? Eat less meat? Participate in Meatless Mondays or Veganuary? If we ask anything less than veganism, should we still tell people that veganism is the endgame and be clear about it?

Let's name what we ask of both individuals and institutions the *call to action*. There's no consensus among vegans about the best call to action. There isn't even consensus about what we've been doing so far. Some activists will blame what they perceive as slow progress on the fact that we have *not* been asking people to go vegan. Others will say the opposite: we've been emphasizing the "Go vegan!" message too much. In any case, many vegans will say our call to action hasn't been ideal. That's all the more reason to take a look at it.

When tackling the question about the call to action, we can again approach it from a pragmatic or idealistic direction. If we're pragmatic, we look for the call to action that has the most bang for the buck, the one that will get us the most results we want (less suffering, killing, or injustice). Those who are more idealistic, on the other hand, will be greatly concerned about what the morally correct question to ask is. Is it, for example, ethically appropriate to ask people to eat less meat, try out veganism for a while, or focus on avoiding fish and chickens first of all?

The question here revolves around whether we can or should use an *incremental* call to action. Incremental calls to action can be formulated differently. The variable can be:

- The frequency (eat less meat; don't eat it during the week, have a vegan day, be vegan before six P.M.)
- The portions (eat smaller portions of meat)
- The period (go vegan in January, as the Veganuary campaign suggests)
- The kind of animals you eat or don't eat (such as, "stop eating chicken," which is the message the organization One Step for Animals suggests)
- The kind of meat (eat more "humane," "free range," "grass fed")

COMPROMISE IS NOT COMPLICITY

Asking something other than what you really want worries many vegans, but it's a common approach among all social movements, and it is one of the hallmarks of pragmatism. In 1806, British abolitionists faced a quandary.[4] For over twenty years, they'd been trying unsuccessfully to outlaw the British slave trade. In the wake of several expensive and humiliating defeats in war and an ongoing conflict with Napoleon's France, the public and political mood for their cause had turned hostile. The abolitionists were growing deeply discouraged. At that dark moment, abolitionist and naval-law expert James Stephen came up with a novel idea. Rather than bringing yet another unrealistic abolitionist bill to Parliament, he thought, why not introduce one that merely made it illegal for British subjects to invest in, insure, supply, or otherwise participate in slave-trading by France and its allies, including notably the United States, and legalize the seizure of French and allied slave ships by British navy vessels and privateers?

This was a genius idea for two reasons. It would play to nationalist sentiments. Naval and maritime interests would love it, as crews would be entitled to claim a percentage of the value of any illegal ship they captured. The British public and politicians didn't realize that roughly two-thirds of British slave ships sailed under either the French or US flag. Although appearing to be patriotic fluff, the bill would dismantle a great deal of Britain's slave trade.

Still, many abolitionists hesitated. Was it right to settle for a partial solution to an absolute evil? Was it possible that by eliminating competition, they might actually wind up strengthening the existing slave trade? And might not the public think the abolitionists were implicitly endorsing slavery conducted under Britain's own flag?

Eventually, the abolitionists decided to follow Stephen's plan. The Foreign Slave Trade Act turned out to be a huge success. It immediately knocked out a large part of Britain's slave trade and, contrary to abolitionist fears, destabilized the rest. *Plus* it reinvigorated support for abolition. Just one year later, the long-sought-after bill ending the slave trade was passed.

This wasn't the only tough compromise the abolitionists made. An even harder one had occurred almost twenty years earlier. At one of their first meetings, they voted to work only on shutting down the slave trade and not on freeing Britain's (and its colonies') slaves. They didn't arrive at that decision lightly. They knew it meant leaving more than half-a-million people enslaved, most in horrific circumstances in the Caribbean sugar fields. However, they considered that battle unwinnable *at that time.* They hoped that eliminating the slave trade would lay the foundation for future emancipation, which it did.

A Lesson from Gluten free

For the members of the British anti-slavery movement, pragmatic demands were instrumental in achieving their final objective. To show how a pragmatic call for action may be similarly beneficial to animal advocates and vegans, we turn to another food-related phenomenon.

Whatever country you're from, you've probably noticed that over the last five or ten years the trend of gluten-free products and meals has ballooned. It hasn't been around for as long as veganism, but gluten-free options in stores and restaurants seem to be even more prominent than vegan ones. How did this happen?

The answer hit me when I saw a woman post a comment on Facebook. She said something like this (Fig. 6):

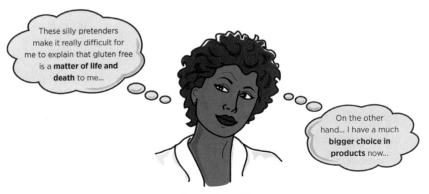

Fig. 6: A Gluten-free Observation

For this woman, being gluten free is a matter of life and death. She suffers from celiac disease, and even a gram of gluten can have serious consequences. On the other hand, there are people who "pretend" they need to be gluten free. They believe that gluten is harmful and that avoiding it has a positive effect on their health and energy levels. Scientists seem to disagree, claiming that for most people without celiac disease avoiding gluten isn't necessary. Let's call these people *pretenders*, although using this term in this context is not meant to imply any disrespect.

As gluten-free pretenders don't need to avoid gluten like the plague, they won't be so strict about it. They might be comfortable with consuming a bit of gluten here and there, perhaps avoiding it only some of the time. The (allergic) woman's complaint was that these pretenders made it more difficult for her to persuade other people—such as waiters in restaurants—to take her special diet as seriously as they should. The waiters and others might be used to dealing with pretenders, assume that our woman with celiac disease is one of them, and thus might not be strict enough in handling her request. Compare this with how vegans find it problematic when some people call themselves vegetarian or vegan, but eat fish now and then or allow other exceptions. These people, we believe, make things harder for the rest of us by creating confusion. Before we know it, we'll receive a fish on our plate in a restaurant because the chef is thinking of the last "vegan" who happily ate it.

What's crucial here is the other point our woman with celiac disease makes. Thanks to all the pretenders, she now can choose among a wealth of gluten-free products, in both stores and restaurants—products that a couple of years ago were simply not available. The parallel should be clear. In the vegan movement, we have a small group of genuine vegans for whom eating vegan food is a matter of life and death, if only in a moral sense. However, a much greater collection of people likes to eat vegetarian or vegan meals now and then, to different degrees. Actually, the numbers more or less coincide for the vegan movement and the gluten-free phenomenon: about one person in a hundred is allergic to gluten or is vegan. The part of the population that wants to reduce their gluten or meat intake is many times larger. One of the reasons there are many more reducers than vegans is of course that being a reducer is, or seems, much easier than being a vegan for most people. And these numbers are highly significant.

WHY MEAT REDUCERS ARE CRUCIAL

The gluten-free pretenders or part-timers have been crucial to the growth of gluten-free products. They helped create a market that suppliers found

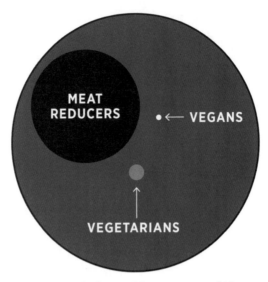

Fig. 7: Meat Reducers, Vegetarians, and Vegans

profitable. In the same fashion, meat reducers are crucial for our own movement. Here are the main reasons:

1. *Many meat reducers together may change the system faster than a few vegans.*

As reducers together consume many more vegetarian and vegan meals than vegetarians and vegans (see Fig. 7), we may assume they are also the main buyers of veg meals and products. It makes sense that producers and distributors of vegan meals and products see this segment of the market as their primary target (Shore). Yves Potvin is the founder and president of the Canadian company Gardein, which produces meat alternatives. In a personal correspondence, he told me: "Flexitarians are the key to changing the world and the largest group that purchases Gardein, as vegans and vegetarians are still a small percentage of the population and flexitarians are on the rise." Likewise, Seth Tibbott, founder and chairman of the famous Tofurky brand, told me: "While vegans and vegetarians both punch above their weight, we estimate that they are at most responsible for around 20 percent to 25 percent of our customer base. We feel that meat reducers, some of whom are former vegans or vegetarians, account for the vast majority of our sales." Even at a niche store like the Herbivorous Butcher in Minneapolis, the owners estimate that 60 to 70 percent of their customers are omnivores or reducers (Bird). The same can probably be said for most vegan restaurants.

This large group of reducers, then, drives demand and has a greater effect on the market than the small group of vegetarians and vegans. Food companies develop new items to meet this demand—sometimes to compensate for their declining sales of animal-based products or as a hedge against the future. Supermarkets will offer these products, and chefs prepare meals with them.[5]

What we see here is a virtuous circle of supply and demand. As demand grows, choices increase and so does the acceptance of eating vegetarian or vegan. This growth makes it easier for everyone to move further along the vegan spectrum, just as the pretenders made shopping, cooking, and eating easier for the woman with celiac disease. Keeping in mind the importance for each of us of vegan alternatives, it's not a stretch to say that many of this book's readers might be vegetarian or vegan right now thanks at least in part to the much greater group of meat reducers who unwittingly prepared the road for them. In short, whereas reducers aren't the embodiment of individual change, they seem crucial for societal change. And societal change, in turn, should lead to more individual change. The Faunalytics report on former vegetarians states: "Farmed animals *may* benefit more from efforts focused on encouraging the many to reduce their animal-product consumption as opposed to inspiring a relatively small fraction to achieve total elimination of animal-based foods" (Asher et al. 2014, p. 3).

Reducers, much less than vegetarians and vegans, are not necessarily motivated by ethical reasons. The motivation, however, is irrelevant in terms of the effect they have on demand. I talk about motivations in the next chapter.

2. *As a group, meat reducers save more animals than vegetarians and vegans.* All the reducers together are responsible for avoiding more animals being killed than vegetarians and vegans combined. (If we would juxtapose

THE CASE OF SOYMILK

Supply and demand is also exemplified in the example of soymilk and other dairy alternatives. Today in the UK, for instance, about one in five households chooses to buy plant-based alternatives for dairy milk. Between 2011 and 2013, the market grew an incredible 155 percent, according to a Mintel study (Harrison-Dunn). Even the most optimistic vegan will know without seeing any polls that this market doesn't consist entirely of vegans, nor are all of these consumers turning to alternatives because they care about what happens to dairy cows and their calves. They use such products mainly for health reasons and taste preferences. These motivations make the market grow, as they lead producers to offer more and better alternatives, which has made it easier for you and me to be vegan today. ■

reducers plus vegetarians against vegans, the difference would be even greater.) A 2016 national poll by the Vegetarian Resource Group in the US shows a total of 3.4 percent vegetarians and vegans versus 33 percent of the population eating vegetarian or vegan meals (VRG). The total number of these meals eaten by reducers (they are broken down according to frequency of vegetarian meals) is about three-to-four times higher than the amount eaten by vegetarians and vegans together.

3. Meat reducers are more likely to go vegetarian or vegan than regular meat eaters.

According to the Faunalytics report *Advocating Meat Reduction and Vegetarianism to Adults in the US*, when compared to regular meat consumers, moderate meat consumers are twice as willing to go vegetarian, while semi-vegetarians are almost six times as willing (2007). Research has shown that so-called small wins—minor victories that people or organizations achieve—are psychologically invaluable, with an effect that is disproportionately greater than the accomplishment itself. Pulitzer Prize–winning journalist Charles Duhigg, who popularized the concept of small wins in his book *The Power of Habit*, writes: "Small wins fuel transformative changes by leveraging tiny advantages into patterns that convince people that bigger achievements are within reach" (p. 112). Asking people to take small steps (going a day without meat, by way of illustration) and thus increasing the chance of an experience of success, is a crucial step for creating change. The opposite is also true. People may feel defeated whenever they reach for something and don't succeed.

In the next chapter, I look closer at some psychological theories that may explain why reducers would make better candidates to go vegetarian or vegan than regular meat eaters.

4. *Less Backsliding*

According to different studies, former vegetarians and vegans are more likely than current ones to have stopped eating meat all at once. People who stayed vegetarian or vegan are more likely to have made a gradual rather than abrupt transition to vegetarianism or veganism. The evidence is still only tentative, but it's something to take into account. The advice to smokers to "cut back before you quit" may well apply to omnivores, too (Haverstock and Forgays, Asher et al. 2014).

5. *The "Spread" Factor*

One final reason why reducers might have more influence is that they're more spread out within society and thus come into contact with more people, institutions, and specific settings upon whom and in which they can exert an influence. The joint requests of the reducers for meals and products will be spread over more and different locations, restaurants, supermarkets, and other outlets.

This way, the reducers potentially confront a more substantial part of the supply with the vegan demand. A restaurateur may also be inclined to make more of an effort for seven people who participate in a Meatless Monday campaign, let's say, than she would catering for one vegan. Apart from the numbers, vegans may be more likely to flock together, preferring vegan restaurants and eating in vegan groups, so their potential influence is reduced. On the other hand, vegans may be publicly more vocal and in that respect affect the environment more completely. For instance, it's usually vegans who, by their writing and communicating, manage to induce a company to remove an animal ingredient from their product and veganize it. This is all somewhat speculative, and it would be interesting to examine the repercussions of the "spread."

IMPROVING OUR CALL TO ACTION

Our ambition to create a better world for animals translates most clearly to a (more or less) vegan world. Since, in general, nonvegan products and consumption habits contribute to the suffering of animals, it would seem inconsistent for vegans to ask for anything less from people than "Go vegan!" Therefore, if consistency in our aims and ideology is the criterion for our call to action, veganism would appear to be the bottom line. However, if we consider effectiveness as the criterion, we should at least include in our outreach a message of *reducing* our consumption of animal products. Reducing consumption isn't as dramatic or hortatory as "Go vegan!" so let's examine criteria that may help us determine and formulate a strong reducetarian call to action.

1. *A Call to Action that People Are Open to*
A call to action should be formulated so that people don't immediately close their eyes and ears to it. We're not talking about implementation, but the step before: people's openness to listen to what vegans are saying, writing, or demonstrating. They'll be more prepared to listen when we ask them something that's feasible and they can imagine themselves doing.

We can, of course, tell them to become vegetarian or vegan, but it's useful to remember that for the largest segment of our audience, such a move is daunting. As I already pointed out, "for most adults . . . eliminating meat seems to be a frightening or absurd notion. Almost 8 in 10 say that they are 'not at all likely' to ever give up eating meat entirely" (Faunalytics 2007)—a number that might have moved slightly in our favor in the last decade. That said, a more recent Belgian poll showed that virtually none of the regular meat eaters had any desire to become a vegetarian (Ivox). And we're not even talking about veganism here.

Whereas the public's view of vegetarianism and veganism seems to have improved in recent years, many people still retain negative associations with vegetarians and especially vegans, as well as with the idea of animal rights (Cooney 2014, p. 48). This obviously doesn't help make the direct appeal to "Go vegan!" more effective.

Of course, we could ask ourselves to what extent our audience's receptivity matters. One reason for the aversion is undoubtedly people's clinging to their preferred diet, and many will always look for an excuse not to pay attention. However, even if we can't entirely control people's willingness to listen, it would nonetheless make sense to choose messages that are more helpful in creating an attitude of openness.

2. A Call to Action that People Actually Follow up on

Although "Go vegan!" may not be the ideal message because it's too difficult an ask, saying "Eat less meat" (or fewer animal products) may not be our most effective option either. For one thing, "Eat less meat" isn't concrete. People won't know what to do or have a clear idea of whether they're accomplishing the goal. Many will say they're *already* eating less meat, but in many cases that may simply not be true.[6] Another concern is that behavioral change—especially when it's about a difficult subject like food, and particularly animal products—is easier when people have some kind of structure or system. In their book *Switch: How to Change Things When Change Is Hard*, Chip and Dan Heath offer the tip to "script the critical moves." They suggest we should give our audience clear instructions about the measures to be taken. This is especially necessary because people otherwise risk incurring so-called analysis paralysis. Confronted by too many options and too much conflicting information, they end up running in mental circles and do nothing.

Assuming we agree it's strategic in many situations not to use the "Go vegan!" call to action but to suggest that people eat less meat or fewer animal products, here is a list of concrete calls to action we *could* use:

- Meatless Monday (or any other meatless day, such as Thursday Veggieday in Belgium or Tuesday in Brazil)
- Vegan before Six, an idea launched by American food blogger and former *New York Times* journalist Mark Bittman
- Weekday vegetarianism
- Home veganism
- A temporary "vegan challenge" or "Veganuary"-type pledge (see box on p. 41)

Each of these calls to action has its advantages and disadvantages. Nonetheless, all provide people with a system or structure to which they can commit. They also may seem more feasible and doable than asking people to go "cold turkey."

A call to action I'm less in favor of is to ask people to eat smaller portions of meat, as many government recommendations would have it. This request isn't concrete, it's hard to establish a campaign around, and most importantly, it won't offer people the opportunity to try out new foods. It's unlikely that meat eaters will have a small cut of beef *and* a piece of tofu or half a veggie burger on their plate. Consequently, this will not bring them any closer to meals *without* meat (or animal products), even if it could obviously have a substantial effect on demand if many people ate this diet.

3. *A Call to Action that Is Credible*
No matter how strong the case for veganism, nonvegans will try to poke holes in the argument, or give reasons why veganism isn't viable. Vegans may not find these objections credible, but the relevant factor here is that those who offer criticisms usually, though not always, believe them. Consider the argument that the vegan diet promotes health. Whether rational and evidence-based claims can be made against vegan diets isn't as important as whether the claims for veganism are credible in the eyes of the public, health professionals (including doctors), and politicians. It's difficult for anyone to find sound reasons for *not* reducing consumption of animal products. Health objections certainly don't apply. Most people

Veganuary and Other Pledge Campaigns

Many vegan organizations around the world run pledge campaigns, wherein one commits to be vegan (or vegetarian) for a period. In terms of our metaphor, people are invited to live for a while in Veganville and see how they like it.

The most well-known example is the Veganuary campaign, which began in the UK (www.veganuary.com). Campaigns like these possess some distinct advantages. Many of those who consider going vegan fear that at some point afterward they might abandon the diet. Thinking merely about future failure, embarrassment, or criticism can prevent these individuals from doing anything at all. In pledging to go vegan for a period, they're not committing to be vegan forever, which is likely instrumental in enabling them to start moving.

Campaigns like Veganuary run not only for a specific number of days, but at a specific time of year. The fact that everyone starts together is itself a great incentive to participate. Those who fear they might not be up to the challenge of a month without animal products can find encouragement in the idea they're not alone, but with thousands of others. Veganuary had nearly 60,000 participants from 150 countries in 2017. This mass participation is comforting and helps to build a norm and maybe even some pressure: *Wow, so many people are doing it! I can't really not do it, can I?* That the campaign begins at a certain point in the year is also a terrific means of garnering media attention. It is a golden opportunity for many restaurants and cafeterias to concentrate their vegetarian or vegan efforts as an experiment for a short period of time. ∎

in the industrialized world eat too much animal protein, and one can't really state (and I've never heard it stated) that reduction is impracticable. Credibility is especially vital when we want to get influencers and institutions onboard. (See chapter 4, regarding institutional change.)

4. A Call to Action that Reduces Suffering and Killing As Much As Possible
Some concrete calls to action that people are likely to follow up on may
not have a substantial impact. You could ask people to stop buying and
eating foie gras. But even if everyone agreed, relatively little would be
achieved since foie gras is a specialty dish not eaten by large numbers
of consumers. One could make a good case for asking people to stop or
reduce eating the animals who are the most numerous victims: chickens
and fish. That said, some easier actions, such as the foie gras campaign,
can be stepping stones toward more comprehensive behavioral change.
This fact is why advocacy against fur or circuses that use animals—which
utilize only a fraction of the number of animals in the meat industry—
can conscientize people about a range of animal advocacy issues.

But What about Vegan?

In chapter 5, I talk more about the concept of veganism and vegan
communication. Here, I'll just touch on the "Go vegan!" message and the
use of the word *vegan*.

I see a reducetarian call to action as complementary to a vegan call to
action. I'm not suggesting we *never* ask people to "Go vegan!" Nor am I
claiming we should never use the word *vegan*, as it is useful and becoming more widely known. What I *do* suggest is we use both "Go vegan!"
and reducetarian messages and select which one to use depending on
our audience. When we're communicating with people at large, we may
consider something other than "Go vegan!" if we're trying to build a critical mass. Josh Tetrick, founder and CEO of Hampton Creek, the company
that wants to take laying hens out of the food chain by developing egg
alternatives, offers the following advice for appealing to the mainstream:
"Never use the word *vegan*" (Choi). Tetrick is talking about mainstreaming vegan products to customers. He's not directly raising awareness; he's
selling a product. He knows that many shoppers think of *vegan* negatively—remember the concerns about taste—and so he avoids it.

In my experience, the "Go vegan!" approach can work with certain
audiences and situations:

STEALTH VEGANISM

What if *not* using the word vegan sells more vegan stuff? Years ago, in a Whole Foods supermarket somewhere in California, I was looking for a vegan cake, which someone told me was sold at the store. I couldn't find it, and asked the person behind the counter where it was. She showed me the cake and said it no longer was marked *vegan*. She said it had been selling three times better since the company altered the label.

Recently, I've seen more and more places that are what I describe as "stealth vegan." This means that the fact that all their products are vegan is communicated subtly, if at all. In Australia, a fast-food chain called Lord of the Fries is vegetarian and vegan, but you have to look hard to notice that in their communication. I was told that most of the chain's clientele don't know they're not eating meat. Las Vegas hosts the famous Ronald's Donuts, a hole-in-the-wall. Nothing on the building betrays anything vegan inside. And if you want to know which donuts are vegan, you have to ask.

If these places don't want to use the word *vegan*, that's obviously because they think or know that the term turns more people off than it attracts. The word to most people doesn't indicate added but subtracted value. To get a sense of how you might feel, compare how you might react to an all-gluten-free restaurant. If you're honest with yourself, you probably imagine those dishes won't be as good as the "regular" ones, and that something (taste, perhaps) was removed from them.

All this will change as the general population's appreciation of vegan products increases. One approach to use to make that appreciation grow may be to let people eat vegan food without telling them so. ■

- Young audiences (especially teenagers) like the black-and-whiteness of the message. For them, the vegan identity may be useful and appealing, a statement of opposition. (See chapter 5 for more on the vegan-identity issue.)

- Students, academics, and intellectuals might be more open than most to consider veganism, speciesism, animal rights philosophy, and other aspects of the human–animal relationship.
- People who already care about the welfare of farmed animals, or are vegetarian or close to it. Vegans can definitely encourage these individuals to take another step.
- One-on-one conversations, where it's possible to tell if someone is genuinely interested in a philosophical debate on the topic of veganism.

Finally, regarding use of the V-word: the nouns (*veganism*, *vegan*, *vegans*) are trickier than the adjective (as in a *vegan* meal). The nouns are binary terms: you are vegan or you're not—or at least, people will retain this impression as long as vegans consider it something black and white. (See chapter 5 for a discussion on this.) You may have no interest in becoming fully vegan, so the noun may not appeal to you. If you're a vegetarian or a part-time vegan, you may feel excluded by the noun *vegan*. You don't belong to that group, and "veganism" doesn't apply to you. The nouns are "exclusive"; they exclude you.

The atmosphere surrounding *vegan* as an adjective in *vegan* meals or *vegan* products is completely different. If you suggest to people they might like to eat a vegan meal or buy a vegan product, you're not asking them to "become a vegan." Everybody can eat a vegan meal or buy a vegan product; you don't need to be a vegan. It's much more inclusive; it *includes* you.

Incidentally, it's worth mentioning that we shouldn't see vegetarianism as so much *less* than veganism. Not only is the word *vegetarian* more palatable to people than *vegan*, but research suggests that the extra impact that vegans make compared to vegetarians may be small. Cooney states in *Veganomics* (p. 12) that "vegetarians do almost as much good for farm animals as vegans. They reduce 88 percent as many days of suffering, and spare 94 percent as many lives" (Cooney, quoting Sethu). In other words, any advocacy to remove those last percentages of

The Radical Flank Effect and the Overton Window

The "radical flank effect" (Haines) describes how more radical groups or parts of a movement can influence how moderate segments are perceived. If my organization asks an individual for something hard, but your organization's ask of that individual is even more difficult, then my request will sound more reasonable to the individual by comparison. Another way to put this is that the more extreme ask may help to shift the so-called Overton window, which is the range of ideas the public will accept or be prepared to discuss. When the frame of that window shifts, the unthinkable can become the possible, or the possible can become policy.

The radical flank effect works both ways, however: radicals may discredit a movement and lead the audience to identify the whole movement with that flank. Think of how the audience might believe the animal rights movement to be radical or even violent because of some actions by the Animal Liberation Front. The frame of the Overton window may then shift in the other direction: complete repression of animal activists may be unthinkable at one moment, but considered sound policy the next. Vegans should, of course, try to ensure the window-frame shifts so that our desired outcomes move toward becoming policy and normative (Bolotsky). ∎

animal consumption—or even for people to switch from vegetarianism to veganism—suffers from diminishing returns.

Objections against a Reducetarian Call to Action

In 2000, I cofounded EVA —Ethical Vegetarian Alternative—in Belgium. EVA was actually established as a vegan organization, and some people wanted the word *vegan* in the name. However, we decided against that for reasons of public acceptability. Several years later, we went a step further (some would say backward), and started to think about a message of reducing animal products rather than total avoidance. Some within our group didn't like the idea at all. I myself had only slowly become more open to the reduction message.

Asking for reduction when we want total avoidance or zero consumption is understandably difficult for many vegan animal advocates to accept—as it was for the abolitionists when they considered James Stephen's idea (see the first part of this chapter). In the following pages I respond to some of the arguments against focusing significant efforts on a reducetarian call to action. Some objections will be grounded in idealism (concerns about rightness), others in pragmatism (concerns about effectiveness).

1. "It's immoral to ask for anything less than vegan."

To ask for anything less than what we truly want, the reasoning goes, is to condone the rest. If we ask people to reduce, we are saying (or could be interpreted as saying) that eating less meat is acceptable. If we ask people to become vegetarians, they might get the impression that consuming eggs and dairy products is morally inconsequential. When we ask people to go vegan incrementally, we're suggesting that people can take their time to phase out animal products from their lives. These incremental-isms are incompatible with the idea that animals have rights. If we agree with this premise, then we can't "allow" these rights to be abnegated, and so it's unacceptable to introduce these rights gradually or partially. From an idealistic position, these are non-negotiable absolutes. The bottom line of this reasoning would be that we must always and unambiguously present veganism as a moral imperative.

To strengthen their case against a reducetarian call to action and illustrate the moral imperative of veganism, some vegan advocates make comparisons with human-related issues. They state, for example, that we'd never tell child-abusers or women-beaters they should hurt their children or spouses less often. Rather, we'd require them to stop entirely, immediately. In this respect, the Meatless Monday campaign is as immoral as a child abuse–free Monday campaign. (Note that Meatfree or Meatless doesn't mean vegan, which is another reason for some to be critical of this campaign.)

Drawing this parallel only makes sense from a strictly theoretical standpoint. Even then it may be a stretch. However, it's almost impossible to maintain the comparison when you realize how different the two situations are in the real world. Whereas almost everyone disapproves of child abuse, almost everyone actively celebrates eating animal products. Child abuse is illegal. Using animals is not only legal, but an "essential" part of our economy and culture. One could object that something is wrong, no matter how many people approve of it or celebrate it. But even if this idealistic view is correct, it misses the point if our focus is on results rather than moral consistency or correctness. Issues with such dramatically different public (including legal and political) support require different strategies, no matter what our truth might be.

By way of illustration, think of how much easier it would be for a vegan restaurant to avoid criticism with a NO FUR ALLOWED sign at the door than with one that stated NO LEATHER ALLOWED. How confrontational or forceful we can be in our actions and communication toward other people is to a large extent determined by public support for what we do. David Palmer, the American dentist who shot Cecil the lion, met with almost universal criticism, and no one who condemned Palmer met with much resistance. Obviously, you can't use the same kind of communication with meat eating, which is supported by almost everyone. The graph on the next page (Fig. 8) makes this clear.

If we really believed that today, in this society, we should condemn eating animal products to the same extent we condemn abusing children or sex trafficking or bonded labor, the implications would be enormous. It would mean physically attempting to stop people from buying or eating animal products, in supermarkets and restaurants, always and everywhere, because that's what you'd do you if you saw someone severely beating a child or torturing a woman or shackling a worker to the desk.

Finally, as the example of the abolitionists illustrates in the domain of human rights campaigns, it's not off-limits to compromise and to ask

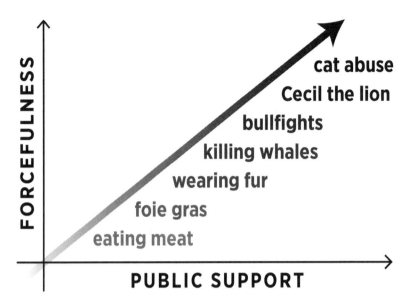

Fig. 8: Forcefulness vs. Public Support

pragmatically for what is possible, rather than what is ideal. Another example of this pragmatism in the face of crisis is found in "Operation Ceasefire" (see box below).

2. "If we ask for reduction, people will just stop at reduction."
One could argue that when people are asked to make small steps, they'll *at best* complete them and stop. Undoubtedly, some may become complacent after undertaking the first steps and go no further. According to the well-established self-perception theory, however, people develop attitudes and beliefs by observing their own behavior. They may perform a

---

OPERATION CEASEFIRE

In 2006, the city of Boston experienced an appallingly high homicide rate among gang members. In an effort to stop the violence, Reverend Jeffrey Brown developed "Operation Ceasefire," which resulted in a drastic decline in casualties. Brown's strategy entailed working with

---

gang leaders and confronting them with concrete consequences, both positive and negative. When Brown talked to one gang leader about stopping the violence, the young man responded that he couldn't just stop "cold turkey." Brown then had an idea: *What about a temporary ceasefire?* Brown writes:

> So we created that between Thanksgiving and New Year's, and we called it season of peace.... I had them in a room, and I made the pitch for the season of peace and asked for their approval. And that's when I got my first indication that this might work, because a young guy gets up, and he says, "All right, so do we stop shooting at midnight on Wednesday night? Or do we stop on Thanksgiving morning? And do we start shooting again on December thirty-first or on January first?"

This wasn't easy for Brown:

> It was a conflict for me, because I was like, "I don't want you to start shooting at all." But I said, "Okay, you stop shooting Wednesday night and you can start again after New Year's Day." Now, you know, ethically I was like, "I can't believe you told them they could start shooting after the first of the year." (Cuddy, p. 83)

But it worked. Despite his hesitation, Brown was trying "to get them to establish peace and give them a sense of what it's like to be able to go into a neighborhood and not have to look over your shoulder every five seconds." In other words, he wanted people to have a certain positive experience, which might motivate them to continue it. (Interestingly, in ancient Greece, a truce temporarily suspended warfare for the duration of the Olympic Games, a practice that was adopted by the modern Olympics.)

It's easy to see the pragmatic value of working with incremental messages and small asks. People find it easier to take smaller steps than larger ones. If we object to incrementalism on idealistic grounds (and I repeat: I think comparisons with human situations are often unproductive and should be made carefully), we may want to think about Jeffrey Brown and his experiment with gangs. Was his strategy immoral? I definitely don't think so. ∎

small action for animals or for their health and start to see themselves as people who care about animals or their health, based on their behavior. This makes it easier for them to take further steps and be open to bigger asks (Freedman and Fraser).

Moreover, research tells us that most people change in stages. Only one in five vegetarians (we're not even talking about vegans) goes from omnivore to vegetarian overnight and two thirds of vegans start as vegetarians. (For an overview of the research, see Cooney 2014, p. 60.) Getting people to take the first step, when so many still have no intention of doing anything at all, is crucial. Any successful experience they have in eating vegetarian or vegan food is therefore significant.

Remember also the gluten-free phenomenon. The point of the reducetarian strategy is that the more reducers there are, the easier it becomes to move further along the vegan spectrum. Even if most reducers would be happy with a couple of meatless days a week, this *in itself* may be enough to lead to the tipping point, so that these same people or their children will be pushed further along the vegan spectrum by changes happening in society as a result of their combined individual changes.

3. "People will reduce anyway when we ask them to go vegan."
If we ask people to go vegan, then at least we're speaking our truth and not betraying our goal or the animals—so the argument goes. There is more chance that people will effectively turn vegan.

As indicated, only a fraction of the general public has any intention of becoming vegans, so we may assume this is not a message that will capture their attention and make them listen. For those who would pay attention, it's possible that they, upon hearing a "Go vegan!" message, won't follow through but may meet us in the middle by reducing consumption. However, this is much more likely if, after our "Go vegan!" message, we explicitly ask people to reduce. This is the "door-in-the-face" technique, where we start with a big ask and follow it with a smaller one. This technique obviously is not about a "Go vegan!" ask, as our final request is reducetarian in nature. Presumably, vegans who object against a reducetarian ask wouldn't want to voice this follow-up.

4. "At least we should be clear that the goal is to go vegan."
Some vegans are open to asking people to reduce, but only in combination with an explicit end-goal. They might say: "Yes, you can reduce, but ultimately the goal is to go vegan and create a vegan world." These people feel strongly about emphasizing moral justice. I talk more about using moral arguments in the next chapter. For now, however, suffice it to say I don't believe we have any moral or other requirement always to communicate this goal. It can even be counterproductive. As a case in point, when trying to influence people in power, explicitly formulating the vegan dream may make us appear naive and not credible.

Some idealists demand that organizations are open and outright when their spokespeople are being interviewed on TV or engaging in a public debate. They want the spokespeople to say loud and clear that they want to end animal agriculture or desire a vegan world. For some organizations and individuals, however, serving the message "straight up" to millions of people or key decision-makers might not be strategic. One also wonders why our opposition seems to have no problem reading our final ambition in our outreach (even when we're sugarcoating it) at the same time as many animal advocates lament that our spokespeople or organizations are obfuscating or even "betraying the animals" (Winslow). To make my point, here is a spokesperson for the National Cattleman's Beef Association in the US:

> Meatfree Monday is a sinister plot to drive farmers and ranchers out of business by convincing Americans that meat is bad for your health and bad for the planet. By asking Americans to stop eating meat on Monday this insidious effort drives the extreme vegan agenda forward with a reasonable sounding request. (Williams 2012)

As far as I know, this is not the intention of the organization behind the Meatfree Monday campaign. But it's largely true for animal rights and vegan organizations who support or engage in this campaign. If the meat industry can see the abolitionist danger of Meatfree Mondays, why can't some parts of our movement?[7]

5. *"The difference between vegans and meat reducers is bigger than just their consumption."*
Compared to vegetarians and reducers, vegans also avoid dairy and eggs and won't implicate themselves in anything that requires the use of animals: no cosmetics tested on animals, no support of entertainment with animals (like circuses or zoos), and other places where animals are exploited. Even then, the added effect of vegans won't outweigh the overall contribution of the reducers (certainly not if we include vegetarians in the reducers' camp, as many vegans would have it).

Another, perhaps more significant difference is that vegans (and vegetarians) are more likely to be activists and make a more substantial impact on others. Still, reducers are significant, too, and nothing prevents them from becoming advocates for animals or for meat reduction. Moreover, the vegan advocacy of the vegan isn't by definition more effective than that of the reducers (see chapter 5).

6. "But I did it overnight! Going vegan is so easy today!"

I already touched on this objection. Vegans shouldn't take themselves as the measure of things (see chapter 5). Veganism is still far from the default option, and in many places people have to work hard to find vegan options. Animal products are still normal, natural, and necessary, and when people consider going vegan at all (something which the great majority never does) many are afraid of all kinds of inconvenience.[8] Also, remember: There's some evidence that those who become vegan overnight have more chance of falling off the wagon. Besides, are *you* sure you became vegan overnight? Vegans can suffer from what we may call "vegan amnesia," almost believing they were always vegans and forgetting that they, too, may have transitioned gradually from omnivorism. And they may have been primed by all kinds of events and influences in their childhood or youth.

Our desire to portray going or being vegan as something easy may also tempt us to downplay the nutritional pitfalls. Dietician Virginia Messina, coauthor of *Vegan for Life*, says: "While we want to present veganism as easy, we really do fail vegans, new vegans in particular, if we don't talk about the important details of nutrition."

Conclusion

I've argued in this chapter that a part of our movement's focus, both in individual and institutional change, should be on an incremental call to action. Just as the British abolitionists weren't afraid of campaigning for something that seemed far from their end goal, so we shouldn't be afraid of pragmatically asking for something less than we eventually want.

We can take inspiration from what happened with gluten free. It became a trend because a lot of "part-timers" or "pretenders" created a demand worth meeting. As supply followed demand, people allergic to gluten (as well as pretenders) suddenly had much more choice, and being gluten free became a lot easier and less daunting. Likewise in our movement, meat reducers, a much larger group than vegans, are crucial drivers of the market. They create demand, and if living as a vegan today is relatively easy, we have to thank the nonvegan reducers.

A large number of people reducing the amount of meat they eat may be the fastest way to tip the system—reaching the point whereby meat becomes a lot more expensive because of lower demand, where subsidies get cut, and plant-based products become much cheaper, better, and more available.

I am unable to identify any strong pragmatic or idealistic arguments against giving a reducetarian call to action its due attention. It has enough going for it that it at least shouldn't be actively opposed, just like proponents of the reducetarian ask shouldn't actively oppose people who like to spread a consistent "Go vegan!" message.

In the next chapter, I examine the arguments animal advocates can use to help people change their attitudes and behavior. Here, too, it is important to be pragmatic. 🌍

3

ARGUMENTS

How Do We Motivate for Change?

"It's easier to act your way into a new way of thinking, than think your way into a new way of acting."—**Jerry Sternin**, *The Power of Positive Deviance*

Our goal in the vegan movement is to get as many people as possible to live with us in Veganville. Presently, they're living comfortably somewhere else. Veganville, as we know, is up a mountain, and people won't get there accidentally. Something needs to happen for them to start the trek. Even if we tell them it's acceptable only to travel part of the journey, they'll still need to have some kind of motivation.

When I wrote about goals earlier, I mentioned vegans' double demand: we want people to demonstrate a certain behavior (not consuming animal products) because of certain beliefs (that animals matter morally).

Just as we can be pragmatic in what we ask people to do (what they eat) so we can be pragmatic about which arguments we use to motivate them. Our commitment to ethical awareness doesn't mean we should insist that people change for the same reasons, or that advocating on the basis of ethical consistency or rigor is the best and fastest avenue to our goal.

MORAL VERSUS NON-MORAL FACTORS

When we examine the different factors that drive change for animals, we can distinguish between the moral and non-moral. Most people who consider themselves part of the vegan movement have ethical reasons for not consuming animal products, usually based on a belief that it's unjust to cause a nonhuman animal to suffer or be killed for food. They may further believe that it's wrong to use animals for entertainment or experimentation based on similar criteria.

In addition to these ethical concerns, vegans may be worried about environmental pollution and animal agriculture's contribution to climate change, as well as how raising animals or crops for feed skews a food system that leaves millions of people hungry. That said, these last two worries may be thought of as "indirect" reasons in the light of many vegans' fundamental belief that animals should not be used instrumentally.

Given these philosophical groundings, it's not surprising that the vegan movement focuses a great deal on using moral arguments to influence attitudes and behavior. The message that it is unethical, or at least morally problematic, to eat or wear animal products takes up considerable space in our pamphlets, newsletters, and magazines, as well as on our websites and social media feeds. Advocates post memes to help people understand the ethical dilemmas posed by their consumption habits (diet and otherwise). We publish books about animal rights theory and discuss morality at our conferences. The words on our signs, slogans, and even from our mouths at demonstrations and protests are couched in the language of an ethical awakening. Day in day out, we communicate moral messages through buttons, bumper stickers, and T-shirts, all of them asking or telling people to stop eating animals.

At the same time, it's an inconvenient truth for many of us in the vegan movement that a significant number of vegetarians and vegans avoid animal products because they believe it's healthy to do so. Some eat vegan food because a partner or other household member does, or animal products are too expensive. Others may even simply not like the taste, texture, look, or smell of animal products.

Some of you might be turning up your noses at or feeling uncomfortable with these motivations, which are devoid of concerns about animals per se. Indeed, you may think these examples aren't about veganism at all, since without the ethical aspect we can't call it *vegan* ("plant-based eating" would be more accurate). You may feel that in order to create

permanent change, an ethical motivation or general behavioral alteration must be present. You may deplore how those who avoid animal food
products for non-moral reasons may not avoid other aspects of animal
use (such as entertainment, clothing, or using other consumer products
that involve animals).

In essence, many vegans place little faith in non-moral arguments
and consider them problematic. Conversely, they believe that moral arguments will lead to lasting change. In this chapter, I argue that neither
view is correct.

OUR MOVEMENT'S FOCUS ON MORAL MESSAGES

Sometimes, vegans take the premium we put on moral messages quite far.
Here are two representative illustrations from social media:

> The only way we will ever achieve what we want to achieve is by
> promulgating a sound and clear moral argument that animals are not
> ours to use. That is the only solid foundation on which our hope for a
> vegan world can lie. This is the only thing that is strategic or pragmatic,
> and certainly the only thing that's just.

> Show [the documentary film] *Earthlings* to everyone, show it in schools,
> and then we will all turn vegan overnight.

Many of us hold an uninvestigated belief that moral arguments cause
the great revolutions in the world. We tend to believe that when humanity made moral progress, change happened first and foremost because a
group of people put forth an ethical case for change and others agreed
with it. By way of illustration, we like to believe that slavery in the
US and UK ended because people no longer accepted that their fellow
human beings should be held in bondage, and that abolition occurred
mainly because the righteous stood against injustice and converted
everyone else.

Here's another example from an online discussion:

> In the past, the majority of the population of the United States, particularly in the Southern states, was in favor of slavery and many plantations in the South even depended on it financially. . . . Just because 99% of the population is in favor of eating animal products and celebrates it does not make it any less morally wrong. Therefore, focus all energies on creating a paradigm shift in the culture—help people to realize that animal exploitation is morally wrong.

Whereas no one could claim that moral outrage was *unimportant* in the ending of slavery, it was neither the only nor the main factor in abolition. For one thing, the industrial revolution helped ensure that human labor became more expensive and less convenient relative to automation. (Even slaves have to be housed and fed, so slavery was never entirely cost-free.) For another, the South didn't simply accede to the argument: it seceded, a bloody civil war ensued, and the South was defeated by the North (where slavery was much less important economically). Norm Phelps writes about this:

> African slavery in America was ended by a war conducted by the United States government and supported by both the general public and the corporate capitalist establishment in the North. This fact is universally known; every high school student is taught it. But it is universally ignored by animal activists committed to agitation as the only valid strategy for animal liberation. (p. 171)

Phelps' comment is intriguing. If he's right—and I think he is—why would so many people ignore the fact that slavery didn't end how they think it did? Apparently, we somehow want or need to believe that revolutions like the abolition of slavery occur because of moral awakening, exclusively or primarily. This thinking exemplifies a tendency among vegan animal advocates to want people to stop exploiting animals *because they care about them.* (Remember the "double demand"?)

Slavery is not the only example of a wrong being ended by a non-moral driver. In 1986, the International Whaling Commission (IWC) declared a moratorium on commercial whaling. The IWC might never have reached its decision if the commercial importance of whaling hadn't diminished significantly since the late nineteenth century. Whales—and sperm whales especially—used to be an important source of energy. Whale oil was extracted and used primarily as fuel for lamps, but also in heating, soap, paint, and other products. Countless numbers of whales were killed for this reason.

In 1849, Abraham Gesner, a Canadian physician and geologist, developed kerosene, a liquid made from coal, bitumen (a form of petrol), and oil shale. Unlike whale oil, kerosene was neither smelly nor dirty. It didn't spoil, and, most importantly, was cheaper to produce than whale oil. As kerosene distilleries popped up everywhere and kerosene was commercialized, demand for whale oil collapsed. (Ironically, kerosene sales themselves collapsed when Thomas Edison commercialized his lightbulb technology.) The whaling industry lasted for a while on sales of whalebone, which was used for corsets and other garments. However, that was soon replaced by other materials, and in the end, the industry declined.

Abraham Gesner obviously hadn't been trying to ban whaling—either for moral or non-moral reasons. Yet the result was the same. The last American whaler left port in 1924 and was brought back the next day (Robbins). How much easier it was, still more than fifty years later, to ban commercial whaling in most countries!

Here's another example of social change, one that didn't rely on technological advances. In 2010, Catalonia, a so-called autonomous region in Spain, banned bullfighting. Animal rights organizations had been using the slogan TORTURE ISN'T CULTURE for years. But moral outrage alone didn't kill off this particular form of animal abuse; the motivation was in part political. Many Catalonian nationalists were happy for a practice they considered traditionally Spanish to disappear. Banning bullfighting was a statement of independence, a symbol of a breach with Spanish culture and customs. These sentiments helped many Catalonians to vote in favor of the ban.[9]

Attendance at bullfights in Catalonia was already low by the time of the vote, and it was mainly an older population that still seemed to enjoy them. People might have stayed away because they were morally queasy about bullfighting, but we shouldn't assume this was the only reason: other forms of entertainment may have been easier to access or more attractive. In any case, when something is neither lucrative nor a significant part of the economy, there will obviously be much less resistance to its abolition.

AWARENESS IS OVERRATED

Clearly, factors other than ethical awakening can play a significant role in ending customs or rejecting ideas that people find reprehensible. Conversely, raising awareness with moral arguments is not sufficient in itself and may work less well than advocates hope or expect. Usually, most activists and changemakers, even when they know better, operate according to the basic idea that when we give people the correct information they'll alter their behavior. In the case of vegans, we believe that if (thanks to our outreach) people realize that the suffering and killing of animals for meat is wrong, they'll draw the obvious conclusion and stop eating animal products.

It's not only activists who think like this. Psychologists have long thought it obvious that attitude influences behavior. However, in their studies, they found out that the link was much weaker than they'd supposed, and was dependent upon many factors (Hewstone et al., Holland et al., Kraus, Wicker).[10] There is now a consensus among social scientists and psychologists that providing information alone doesn't change people's behavior: this is the attitude–behavior gap. If we can get beyond the barrier of people not listening to or hearing us, if we can reach them amid all the hundreds of other messages that are fired at them daily, they *may*—in a best-case scenario—get our message and believe it is true and right. But that won't necessarily incite them to real action, which in the end is necessary for there to be an actual impact.

One example of this attitude–behavior gap is offered by philosophy professor Eric Schwitzgebel, who has conducted research into the behavior of ethics professors (Schwitzgebel and Rust). Schwitzgebel found that these individuals—who might be thought to be highly motivated to be ethically consistent or knowledgeable about moral codes and consequences—didn't behave any differently from other professors. Nor did they live more in accordance with their beliefs than others. Schwitzgebel even examined the topic that interests us: eating meat. Whereas ethics professors were much more likely to agree that it was wrong to eat the meat of mammals regularly (60 percent, compared to 45 percent of non-ethicist professors, and 19 percent of professors outside moral philosophy), there weren't any more vegetarians among the ethics professors. Schwitzgebel puts it thus:

> An ethicist philosopher considers whether it's morally permissible to eat the meat of factory-farmed mammals. She reads Peter Singer [moral philosopher and author of *Animal Liberation*]. She reads objections and replies to Singer. She concludes that it is in fact morally bad to eat meat. She presents the material in her applied ethics class. Maybe she even writes on the issue. However, instead of changing her behavior to match her new moral opinions, she retains her old behavior. She teaches Singer's defense of vegetarianism, both outwardly and inwardly endorsing it, and then proceeds to the university cafeteria for a cheeseburger (perhaps feeling somewhat bad about doing so). (Schwitzgebel)

These professors were "morally opposed but not behaviorally opposed to eating meat" (Herzog, p. 201). For vegetarians and vegans, it's easy and tempting to judge these people as hypocritical, weak-willed, or mendacious. However, rather than seeing them as uncaring or selfish, it might be more helpful to examine what trouble or inconvenience they go through, or *fear* they may have to overcome, to maintain ethical consistency.

At this point, people such as our meat-eating ethics professors may experience what is called cognitive dissonance (Festinger), when a value or belief ("I care about animals") and a behavior ("I'm eating animals") contradict one another. (The conflict can also be between different values, beliefs, or ideas.) This dissonance is by definition unpleasant, and we want to avoid it. We have several options: these are so-called "dissonance reducing strategies" (Rothgerber). A few people will resolve the feeling of discomfort by aligning their behavior with their values or beliefs: they become vegetarian or vegan. Most people, however, are wary of changing their behavior, at least when it causes significant inconvenience, and solve the dissonance by doing the opposite: they try to change their beliefs so they're in line with their behavior (eating meat). People attempt, sometimes successfully, to believe in lies and half-truths as rationalizations: "the animals die a quick death," "they are raised for meat," "they don't feel as much as we do," "we need to eat meat," and on through the various "N's" of justification.

A third method by which we deal with the discomfort is by doing what we can to avoid the confrontation with the most uncomfortable parts or implications of our behavior. James Serpell talks about so-called distancing devices. We detach ourselves from the animals we eat and avoid emotional intimacy with them. We conceal factory farms and slaughterhouses. We misrepresent animals in order to make exploiting them easier (Serpell). Or we may, simply, try to ignore the problem and pretend that we're not aware of it—something the literature calls "affected ignorance" (Williams 2008).

ATTITUDE CHANGE CAN FOLLOW BEHAVIORAL CHANGE

Changing our beliefs obviously *can* lead to an alteration in behavior: the link is simply weaker than one would expect. However, vegans tend to overlook the obvious reality that change can work the other way around: altering behaviors can lead to a change in attitude, as Fig. 9 on the opposite page illustrates.

The late Yale University psychologist Robert Abelson notes: "We are very well trained and very good at finding reasons for what we do, but not very good at doing what we find reasons for" (p. 25). Let's look at a couple of examples to see more clearly how someone's behavior can influence their attitudes and beliefs about it.

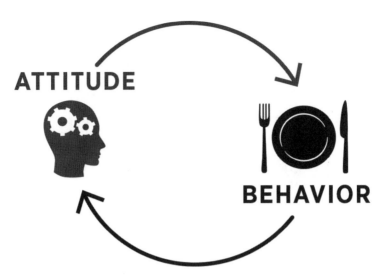

Fig. 9: Two Starting Points for Change

When a democratic government implements a new law, it's usually the case that enough public support exists for it to pass. However, there will always be people (sometimes a large number of them) who don't support the law. Yet, by definition, if the law applies to them, they have to obey it or risk being penalized. This forced behavioral change, however, may be followed by a change in attitude later, so that people who were initially opposed to the law eventually come to accept it.

A classic example is the law on buckling your seat belt. Polls show that many of those who initially opposed wearing seat belts later supported mandatory use (Fhaner and Hane). I can imagine the same switch with the prohibition of smoking in public places. Initially, the ban caused opposition and outrage in many countries. Today, many people can hardly believe or even remember that smoking used to be acceptable in universities or hospitals, or that teachers could smoke at school. Many of those same resisters find it obvious and good that the law was changed.

Here is another example of attitude change being a consequence of behavior instead of the other way around.

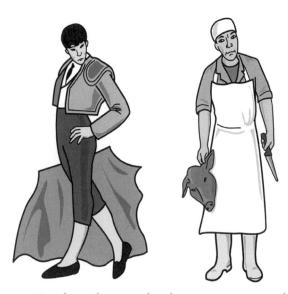

Fig. 10: Who is the general audience most angry with?

Imagine a bullfighter and a slaughterhouse worker (Fig. 10). They both kill bovines for a living, and yet our reaction to their jobs may be entirely different. Most of us will be angrier at the bullfighter's actions than at the slaughterer's. Why? It might be that bullfighting is seen as entertainment and frivolous, whereas many believe that killing cows for food is a necessity—even though, in the final analysis, eating meat is no less trivial than entertainment. Bullfighting also happens in the open, whereas the public can't witness the butchering of animals.

A more fundamental reason why people might judge bullfighters more severely is that (outside of some countries) few of us participate in the "sport," which makes it a lot easier for us to condemn it. Most of us, however, do eat meat, and it's a lot harder to condemn a behavior you're indulging or complicit in. In other words, where you stand depends on where you sit. As long as we eat meat, we are steakholders. Our dependence on meat is so great that it almost prohibits us from thinking rationally about it. It makes us think, as it were, with our stomachs.

Another example of how our behavior influences our beliefs and attitudes can be found in the study, interestingly titled "The Role of Meat

Consumption in the Denial of Moral Status and Mind to Meat Animals" (Loughnan et al.). Participants had to indicate, by means of a questionnaire, their moral concern for animals, and judge the moral status and mental states of a cow. Here's the catch: The researchers served half the participants dried beef, whereas the remainder received nuts. The researchers observed that eating meat reduced the perceived obligation to care for animals and the perceived moral status of the cow. Moreover, those who'd been served meat were less likely to ascribe to the animals the mental states necessary to experience suffering. The researchers concluded:

> The current study provides direct evidence that eating meat leads people to withdraw moral concern from both animals in general and the animal they ate. . . . Meat eating appears to have an important impact on the perception of meat animals, which are viewed as unworthy of moral consideration and lacking the mental states necessary to experience suffering. (Loughnan et al.)

It's easy to imagine that this dynamic not only occurs in individuals but at the level of society and culture: we don't eat animals because we consider them inferior, but we consider them inferior because we eat them, and have been doing so for a long time. Seeing animals like this is one more strategy to reduce unpleasant (dissonant) emotions.

Here's an example of behavior influencing attitudes of an altogether different kind. In October 2016, the podcast Radiolab ran an episode called "Alpha Gal," featuring Amy Pearl, herself a digital-radio producer. Pearl related how, after she became violently sick when she ate meat, it became clear she'd developed an allergy to a sugar called alpha galactose (alpha gal for short), which is present in the blood of mammals and consequently in red meat. It turned out that the trigger for this sudden allergy was a tick, which has been producing the same effect among hundreds of people.

Amy explains how she'd always been into meat. Meatballs were her favorite dish and she loved to eat at steakhouses. Becoming suddenly allergic to (red) meat was not fun for her, and for a while she fought it. She even landed in the hospital emergency room after stubbornly attempting a few bites of grilled steak during barbecue season. However, the episode ends with Amy saying how she feels about eating meat now:

> I don't think I would go back to eating meat necessarily. . . . I wish I could be a vegetarian for ethical reasons. . . . It's the factory farming and that kind of stuff. . . . Of course, I'm *forced* to not eat it, but at the same time if I had the willpower I would probably go that way anyway. Also, I think it's great: we're all evolving to be on this planet which is getting harder to be on, and we know that meat takes a lot of resources and now I'm not doing that. So the tick is helping me evolve into a better human being. (McEwen and Kielty)

The tick was the trigger for Amy's behavior change. Her forced behavior change made her more open to the benefits of not eating meat and clearly affected her attitudes.

One final example of behavior influencing or preceding beliefs is the most relevant for our purposes. A significant number of people who start out reducing or avoiding meat and other animal products for health reasons will progress to include ethical reasons for their behavior. In this case, the change starts with a certain non-moral attitude (concern for health), which leads to behavioral change (eating differently), which appears to open the gate for changing attitudes about animals. According to one study, about 25 percent of vegetarians who became vegan for health reasons listed ethical reasons as their current motivation (Hoffman et al., p. 142). Another researcher writes about changing motivations: "Very often health-oriented vegetarians had come to accept the ethical arguments against eating meat or had simply come to dislike it" (Hamilton, p. 160). Anecdotally, you may know vegans in your life, or even be one of them yourself, who stopped eating animal products because they were concerned about their health—either in general or for an acute situation like a heart condition—but then became convinced of the ethical arguments (see also Cooney 2014, pp. 74–75).

What exactly happens when a change in behavior leads to a change in attitude? As we've already seen, the theory of cognitive dissonance may provide part of the answer. In this case, the dissonance-reducing strategy consists of people changing their attitudes so they match their behavior. By way of illustration, when people are legally obligated to wear the seat belt and don't like doing so, their only recourse to lift the dissonance is to start to agree with the idea. Another possible explanation is that when people behave in a certain manner, for whatever or even for no reason, they may realize this behavior is not as complicated or inconvenient as they'd expected it would be. This makes it a lot easier for them to see the benefits of the new behavior, such as how wearing a seat belt makes you safer.

Let's transfer this to the domain of veganism. When people actually listen to vegans' moral arguments (and often we don't even achieve that level of engagement), they know that if they take those arguments and themselves seriously they'll need to change their behavior. But changing their behavior is not something they look forward to doing, because of the inconveniences they fear they'll face, and because they worry they won't be able to enjoy good food anymore. (You may have heard people say they don't want to watch *Earthlings* because they know they'll have to go vegan afterward.) Once they experience that the behavior (eating

MOTIVATED REASONING; OR, WHY FACTS DON'T CHANGE OUR MINDS

From what we've seen so far in this book, you may rightly conclude that the value of rational arguments and facts is relative. Not only do they have to combat age-old ideas and desires, but our minds, vegan or not, are prone to all kinds of illusions, errors, biases, and other conditional responses that prevent us from thinking straight. In many or most cases, people don't seem to seek out rational arguments in order to find out the truth about something, but rather the other way around: they use them to defend the ideas or intuitions they already possess. It seems that our ability to reason developed as a means of justifying ourselves and connect to other people, rather than as a truth-finding instrument (Haidt). "Reason developed not to enable us to solve abstract, logical problems or even to help us draw conclusions from unfamiliar data; rather, it developed to resolve the problems posed by living in collaborative groups" (Kolbert).

What's going on in our heads a lot of the time is what psychologists call "motivated reasoning": our mind is looking for justifications or rationalizations for our intuitions or behavior. Rather than being open to the full range of evidence, most often we want the conclusion of our thinking to be that we don't need to do or change anything. So we recruit reasons and thoughts that justify our favored conclusions. When we're in a "motivated state," we're driven in a certain direction. We're personally involved, and we'll steer our reasoning so it can justify our preferences—preferences that are shaped by our habits and appetites.

Motivated reasoning is neither rational nor objective, and it often has problematic consequences. When people are in a motivated state, they may avoid or discount inconvenient information—also known as facts—which otherwise would be relevant. In one study (Piazza and Loughnan), researchers confronted participants with an imaginary, newly discovered animal species on another planet: "trablans." When the trablans were described as intelligent, people were more morally concerned about the animals than when they were presented as not so smart. However, things got really interesting when, in another study, pigs and tapirs were also presented as intelligent animals. In the case of pigs, which—unlike the tapir and the trablans—people eat, porcine intelligence had much less effect on people's moral concerns for them. In other words, the fact of the pigs' intelligence was strategically ignored. As you will have guessed, it's behavior influencing attitudes again. ∎

vegan meals) isn't so hard and can even be enjoyable, defenses may drop, openness to moral arguments may increase, and compassion can grow. All of a sudden, the idea of animal rights becomes a lot easier to accept. The truth is no longer that threatening.

Self-perception theory, which we already came across, may also help explain what happens when behavior influences attitude. The theory maintains that people may develop their attitudes about something by observing their own behavior. If it were, for instance, to become profoundly inconvenient and expensive to eat animals, people would eat fewer of them and start to think of themselves as the sort of person who eats little or no meat. They'd even be likely to come up with stories about how they'd wanted to eat fewer animals all along. In other words, we may stand up for what we believe, but we may also come to believe in what we stand up for (Meyers, p. 116).

Takeaway One: Allowing All Reasons

This chapter has contained bad and good news. The bad news is something advocates for many causes have probably been aware of for some time but have refused to face head on: awareness is overrated. The good news is that change can also start with behavior, and that people can start caring about animals as a result of a change in behavior for other reasons.

Let's combine these insights with what we know from the previous chapter, and look at the concrete implications for vegan and animal rights advocacy.

The first takeaway is this: We can use whatever non-moral argument can help people change their behavior. Health, environmental, and other arguments can be perfect motivations for people to start moving along the vegan spectrum or to go vegan. We should expect openness to moral arguments to be much greater once people have commenced a certain change in behavior.

These non-moral arguments grow more important when we take into account what we concluded from the preceding chapter: that creating a substantial group of reducers may be the quickest means to change the system. The conclusion from both chapters is that it's vital to use motivations that can get many people to reduce their meat consumption. Health concerns are the main reasons reducers cut back on meat (Cooney 2014, p. 76). Others include the environment and a desire for variation and to try new things. Worries over animal welfare are not top of mind for reducers (Faunalytics 2007).

In the end, we *will* need people to care about animals. Our use and abuse of animals is one of the gravest moral outrages of our time. We want to raise awareness and make people see nonhuman creatures as individuals that should *not* be exploited. To many vegans, any message that downplays this idea is problematic because it doesn't appear to lead to that ethical concern. The same vegans would insist that if we don't communicate the moral gravity of the situation, people will never understand the underlying dynamics of power and exploitation that make that abuse possible. As long as people haven't appreciated this situation, such vegans will argue, they will always reproduce new kinds of injustice.

My point is that, although I agree that animal advocacy needs people who have changed not just in their behavior but also in their hearts and minds, this conscientization doesn't necessarily need to be the starting point, just as the initial motivation for people to start the trek to Veganville isn't that significant. In certain circumstances—depending on the situation, the medium, or the target audience—we can or should move the message about animal ethics to the background or sometimes even ignore it altogether. We can let people experience vegan food for whatever reason, or even for no reason at all.

In vegans' quest for a new kind of person—a *Homo empathicus*, so to speak—it's OK if people's new ethics *follow* their behavioral change rather than *precede* or cause it. It's a mechanism we should be open to and explore and use more in our movement. Not only do the animals not care about what kind of vegans we are but, more importantly, everyone starting out for whatever reason may become the "right" kind of vegan.

Employing the health, taste, environmental, and other arguments is not only acceptable but also commendable. Using a variety of reasons will provide us with more chance of appealing to everyone, including those for whom concern for animals is not strong enough to change their attitudes or behavior. It's always smarter to tag our message onto values that people already possess, rather than tell them which values they *should* have, which mostly means insisting on them having *our* values.

One additional reason for not overemphasizing moral arguments is that apart from this not always being effective, it can also backfire. People have persuasion-resistance; they don't like other people to preach to them. One study on attitudes toward vegetarians shows that vegetarians were rated less positively after respondents imagined their moral judgment of meat eaters. According to the authors, their studies "empirically document the backlash reported by moral minorities and trace it back to resentment by the mainstream against feeling morally judged" (Minson and Monin).

Moreover, when we ask people to change their beliefs and accept our ideology, they will see the change as much greater than their behavior or concerns about their health. Researcher Hank Rothgerber indicates that ethical vegans cause more dissonance-reducing strategies than vegans who argue for protecting one's health. I talk about some of the psychological aspects of communication and persuasion in chapter 5. For now, it's instructive to remember that moral advocacy has downsides, and this gives us one more reason to appreciate other motivations.

COUNTERARGUMENTS

Although I don't suggest at all that we drop moral arguments, I'm aware that people may have concerns or doubts about downplaying them or focusing on other arguments. Let's look at some objections.

1. Does the health argument lead to more chickens and fish suffering?
Some vegans—among whom are those I respect greatly and am usually in agreement with—feel we should only use arguments about animals (killing, suffering, justice, or any combination thereof). The other arguments, they believe, could backfire and, in the short or long term, not have

the desired effect. Their most common concern is that, as the raising of chickens or catching of fish is not viewed as being as ecologically destructive or unhealthy as rearing cows to consume red meat, using environmental and health arguments may cause people simply to shift from eating red meat to eating chickens and fish. (Unlike cows, chickens don't produce greenhouse gases through enteric fermentation. They provide a relatively efficient feed-to-food conversion ratio.) The switch in diet, the argument goes, would mean more animal suffering, as you need hundreds of those smaller animals to provide the flesh equivalent of one cow. I agree that this is a genuine concern and that we should watch out for this "substitution effect," but allow me to suggest a few things to consider.

First, studies and polls aren't at all clear that reducers of red meat will eat more chicken. A 2014 study by The Humane League suggests that red-meat reducers and avoiders actually eat significantly *less* chicken and only marginally more fish than people on a standard diet (Humane League Labs, p. 5). The Faunalytics study that examined lapsed vegetarians found that, among this group, those who avoided beef and/or pork did not consume more fish or chicken (Asher et al. 2016a). Looking at several studies, Nick Cooney also concludes: "It appears that people who cut red meat out of their diet do not end up eating more animals" (2014, p. 110). On the other hand, Matt Ball in *The Accidental Activist* (pp. 188–89) cites several sources that suggest there *is* a shift from red meat to chicken. So we need to conclude that the jury is still out at the moment on this issue.

Secondly, we might want to view people's decisions to switch from eating red meat to chicken or fish over the longer term. Far from being a hard-and-fast commitment to eating animals, omnivores' immediate increase of chicken or fish consumption may be one step along a continuum as they start to include more plants in their diet. Progress is not always linear. One can imagine, as a case in point, that children of health-conscious parents (who may consume fewer cows and pigs but more chickens and fish than the average omnivore) may be more likely to go vegan than the children of average omnivores.

Thirdly, for now, health and environmental organizations *are* talking about shifting from red meat to chicken and fish *anyway*. It is important for our movement to take charge of the health and environmental arguments as much as we can, and frame them also to benefit birds and fish. Nothing should keep us from using health and animal arguments together. When in some contexts and for some audiences we emphasize the health and environmental arguments, we can always also talk about our concerns for the suffering and killing of chickens and fish. We can effectively communicate our issues, saying it's not just a matter of *our* health, but also of *their* lives.

What we should definitely *not* do is to valorize the animal argument as the correct, altruistic argument and denigrate the health argument as "selfish." There's nothing wrong with wanting to maintain wellness; indeed, it might allow us to have more energy to help others. Also, the arguments can intersect. Many animals in factory farms become sick because of the confined and crowded conditions they're bred in, and those diseases (*E. coli*, *Campylobacter*, salmonella, avian flu, and others) may pose a direct threat to humans.

Another, altogether different concern with the health argument is that some vegans exaggerate the health benefits, suggesting a vegan diet is a miracle cure against all illness (including heart disease, obesity, or diabetes) or even the easiest regimen to meet all nutritional needs. Vegan diets do have proven health advantages, and dieticians such as Brenda Davis, Virginia Messina, Vesanto Melina, and Jack Norris provide informative and solid science to back those advantages up. However, it's better not to exaggerate claims about veganism—a tendency I call "vegalomania"—if only to reduce dropout from those who fail to undergo the wondrous transformation they think vegans promised them.

2. Are non-moral arguments less sticky?

As I mentioned earlier, an extensive 2014 study conducted by Faunalytics shows that in the US, 84 percent of vegetarians and vegans stops being vegetarian or vegan at some point. When we only look at vegans, the dropout number is still 70 percent (Asher et al. 2014). I will talk about how to prevent or reduce dropout in more detail in the final chapter of this book. Here, I will briefly discuss how the rate might be related to non-moral motivations.

Among respondents to the study, a majority of current vegetarians and vegans (68 percent) checked "animal protection" as a reason to be vegetarian or vegan, this compared to only slightly more than a quarter (27 percent) of lapsed vegetarians and vegans. In contrast, health motivations were cited by a similar portion of current (69 percent) and lapsed (58 percent) vegetarians and vegans. Although this study can only speak to correlations with lapsing (as opposed to causation) and there are limitations with self-reported data of this nature, the difference in animal-protection motivations is noteworthy and could potentially be suggestive that ethical motivations provide more "staying power" than health motivations.

A conclusion that some people take away from this survey is that protecting one's health is not a good argument to communicate in our vegan outreach and that we should always advocate with moral arguments. I definitely disagree with this conclusion.

If we *had* to pick only one argument, it's clear the ethical one has the most staying power. It is actually the only motivation for being one hundred percent vegetarian or vegan. However, even among those study participants who checked animals as their motivation, no less than 70 percent returned to omnivorism, admittedly from a tiny sample. This number is significantly less than the 95 percent of vegetarians or vegans who said they were only motivated by health reasons, but it shows that animal reasons are not sufficient either. Nick Cooney, based on his overview of other studies, concludes that whereas it's possible ethical vegetarians and vegans stick to their diet longer, the difference doesn't seem too large (2014, p. 91).

More significantly, these numbers don't prove that the health argument is damaging or useless. The authors of the report write: "While the health motivations are associated with a greater degree of lapsing, it is also of note that more people reported these health motivations, suggesting that even if this messaging leads to more lapses, health-related messages may still be helpful in encouraging more individuals to *start* the diet" (Asher et al. 2016a). What if health motivations and health communication were more suitable for attracting many people initially, who might then develop over time into ethical vegans? As stated, indications are that a significant number of health vegetarians may grow to being ethical vegetarians over time.

It's also quite possible that in answering the question about motivations in retrospect, lapsed vegetarians and vegans downplayed their former motivations, or that current vegetarians/vegans identified more motivations than they initially possessed. As Cooney suggests, "Regardless of how much people cared about animals when they were vegetarian, people who have gone back to eating meat will be likely to say they care less about animals" (2014, p. 89). This, again, is explained by the theory of cognitive dissonance.

From the present research, we cannot conclude that health is significantly less sticky a motivation, and more studies are necessary. To suggest dispensing with the health argument, as some people do, seems unwise based on what we know today. The Faunalytics researchers conclude: "The majority of those who adhere to a vegetarian/vegan diet—or have done in the past—have multiple reasons for doing so" (Asher et al. 2016a).

As a side note, the fact that so many people drop out is not as depressing as it may sound to vegans. First, it means the potential for the number of vegans to increase is a lot greater than the present one or two percent. Secondly, many former vegans/vegetarians are interested in picking the diet up again. According to one study, only a minority of ex-vegetarians or vegans said they were now regular meat eaters (Haverstock and Forgays). The average former vegetarian or vegan may be thought of as a meat reducer or even a semi-vegetarian (Asher et al. 2016a), and by now we know how crucial these are. Even if health vegetarians don't stick to their diet consistently but stick *mostly* to it, *and* we could easily "make" more health vegetarians, this argument would favor promoting the health benefits (Asher et al. 2014).

Thirdly, in the same study, more than a third (37 percent) of former vegetarians/vegans indicated that they were interested in resuming a vegetarian/vegan diet. Of these individuals, more than half (59 percent) said they were likely or very likely to do so. Health seems the number-one motivator for re-adopting the diet among those who expressed an interest. Finally, at the least, during the years they were vegetarian or vegan these ex-vegetarians influenced the market, helped create more options by increasing demand, and spared quite a few animals from a life of suffering. Animal Charity Evaluators (ACE) believe seven years to be the strongest estimate we have for the mean length of time vegetarians stay vegetarian.

Takeaway Two: Make It Easier

Our first takeaway was that we should allow for, and work with, all possible motivations, including health, sustainability, and taste, so that people start eating differently. The second takeaway is that, bypassing arguments and motivations, we should also focus on creating an environment that facilitates behavioral change, which in turn can facilitate an alteration in attitude.

It's tempting to think we've come far enough in vegan awareness and product development that it's easy for almost anyone to be vegan by choice. That, however, would be wishful thinking. For many, the taste of many animal-product alternatives (such as cheese, steaks, or salmon) is not on a par with the originals, nor is their availability. It's certainly becoming easier every day for vegans to find their favorite products, but it would be a stretch to say there's ample choice of great products and dishes everywhere. Apart from supermarkets, depending on the country or city you live in, many restaurants and canteens lack a decent vegan option, let alone an acceptable choice. Price can be an issue, too. Meat alternatives, and many fruits and vegetables (especially fresh ones), are more expensive than meat.

Convenience is another factor. People still think they don't know how to use some of these products, or are unsure about which to buy or include in their meals to meet nutritional needs.

Summarizing, we can say that the vegan option is far from being the default.

To see more clearly how alternatives and motivations relate, consider plane flights. Flying is one of the most significant greenhouse-gas generators. Climate change obviously threatens many sentient creatures and even whole species. Imagine that for your job, your mission, or your family, you *need* to be on other continents on a regular basis. The alternatives—traveling over land and/or sea—aren't possible or, because they take much more time, are impractical. In order for you to choose these alternatives, you need to be extremely motivated. Conversely, the better the alternatives are (imagine a superfast and less polluting boat, let's say), the less motivation you need.

Let's bring this to our own domain. Imagine that the only vegan food you could eat for the rest of your (probably curtailed) life was water and bread. Would you remain a vegan? Maybe your answer is a resounding *Yes!* But would you have gone vegan if they had been the *only* possibility? You may shout *Yes!* again, but it's hard to know for sure because we assume your beliefs were influenced by the availability or lack of good alternatives. Likewise, many people today will become vegan as soon as it's easy enough for them. Maybe they'll only start moving when alternatives are everywhere and are as real as the real thing. Maybe they'll need something that's entirely identical, like *clean* meat, a cell culture–based food about which I write in the next chapter. The point is, the simpler we make it to switch, the more people will do so. Hence, we need to move from this situation (Fig. 11):

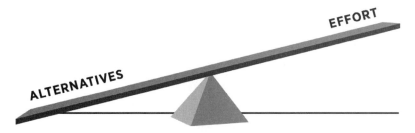

Fig. 11: Lower availability requires more effort.

to this situation (Fig. 12):

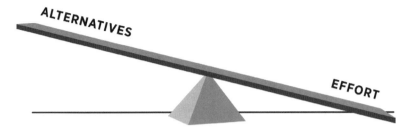

Fig. 12: Higher availability reduces the required effort.

In marketing terms, we could speak about *high switching costs*—the costs one incurs when changing products, suppliers, and brands. The costs can be financial, but they can also be consumers of time or mental space. Phone or insurance companies, for example, want to make switching to their product as easy as possible while at the same time making it difficult to move *from* their product.

In our metaphor, if the road to Veganville offers people everything they need, it will be much easier to start on that road. If people know that every few miles they can get water or find hearty food, a resting place, a place to fix their shoes, it will be much easier to induce them to make the trip. This is the subject of the next chapter.

Conclusion

We've covered a lot of ground in this chapter. Let me recapitulate.

The significance and weight of moral arguments as a driver for change are relative. We want people to be vegan because they care about animals, and we have to raise people's moral consciousness if we seek lasting change. But this concern for animals can come as a result of a change of behavior for other reasons. It's a more indirect route, but if it works, we should use it.

In *Rules for Radicals*, Saul Alinsky writes:

With very rare exceptions, the right things are done for the wrong reasons. It is futile to demand that men [sic] do the right thing for the right reason—this is a fight with a windmill. The organizer should know and accept that the right reason is only introduced as a moral rationalization after the right end has been achieved, although it may have been achieved for the wrong reason—therefore he should search for and use the wrong reasons to achieve the right goals. (p. 76)

This is not a betrayal of the animals. Put succinctly, it's not because we don't talk about things such as ethics and justice that we're not working on them. David Benzaquen, founder of the vegan consultancy company Plantbased Solutions, says: "We are entirely committed to advancing plant-based products that align with our values, but we do not *market* them based on these values" (Leenaert 2017). (See box on p. 92.)

Making Meat Consumption Harder

How easy it is to be vegetarian or vegan is also relative to how easy or difficult it is to be a nonvegan. Apart from making vegan food easier to find, we can try to make it **harder** to produce and consume nonvegan foods. Certain regulations regarding the raising of animals (such as requiring them to have more space) can make production more costly and thus the final product more expensive. For that reason, animal welfare reforms, which by definition offend absolutist animal rights advocates, might, quietly but relentlessly, undermine the economic structure of scale that enables factory farming to survive.

Industrial animal agriculture is doing what it can to make things more difficult for developers of plant-based alternatives. Egg producers in the US, for instance, attempted to make it illegal for Hampton Creek to call its plant-based dip **mayonnaise**. It didn't work, and Unilever is now marketing its own vegan mayo to compete. The dairy industry in Europe was more successful in ensuring plant-based milks couldn't be called **milk**; and plant-based dairy alternatives are taxed more heavily than animal-based dairy products. Lobbying to create a level playing field would be highly valuable here. ■

I listed two important takeaways from the behavior–attitude dynamic. One is that we should use all reasons in our advocacy, particularly those that motivate many people to reduce—as a large group of reducers can change the system the fastest. The other is that we can forget about arguments entirely and focus on people's environment instead. Creating a facilitating environment is what the next chapter is all about. ☺

4

ENVIRONMENT

Making Things Easier

"The way we change [the system] isn't by convincing people to do the right thing. The way we change it is by creating an entirely different system. . . . Hampton Creek is about a philosophy, that believes the only way the good thing wins, is when the good thing is so obscenely better than the not-so-good thing, you cannot help but *do* it."—**Josh Tetrick**, CEO, Hampton Creek

I've talked about the call to action and the arguments we can provide people to start the trip to Veganville. I've said that, as attitude change can follow behavioral change, we should use any motivation that can lead to the latter. I've argued that we need to create an environment that facilitates behavioral change. I abbreviate this last principle to CAFE, which stands for **C**reating **A F**acilitating **E**nvironment. In terms of Veganville: How accommodating is the road? Can travelers find everything they need on the journey: food, water, resting places? How many fellow travelers are there?

By "environment" I mean everything external to the people who want (or whom vegans want) to change. When we create a facilitating environment, the right thing to do becomes the easy thing to do, sometimes to the extent that hardly any effort or motivation is required. For example, we can try to persuade people that classic lightbulbs are bad for the environment or simply make it much more difficult for consumers to buy them since they are, let's say, more expensive or the alternatives are otherwise superior. One obvious means of changing the environment is through legislation. In this case, classic lightbulbs are forbidden by law in Europe and are simply not an option anymore.

Another, classic example of changing the environment is provided by Brian Wansink, a professor of consumer behavior and nutritional science. In his experiment, moviegoers received popcorn in either a large or a small container. Those who received the large container ate 45 percent more popcorn (and 33 percent more when the popcorn was purposely stale!) than those with the small container. Portion size is an element of the environment: small portions can make people eat less without them needing to try to control themselves (Wansink and Kim).

I've actually already mentioned one method of creating a facilitating environment: in chapter 2, we saw that meat reducers, by influencing supply and demand, substantially alter the environment that facilitates change and make it easier for everyone to move along the vegan spectrum. This is an indirect, bottom–up approach to tweaking the environment, but there are more direct methods. Obviously, a reciprocal relationship exists between supply and demand, and we can stimulate or support the supply (production) side more directly, so that demand follows. In addition, we can work with institutions to help us implement change in a top–down direction.

This chapter focuses on the alternatives and the companies that create them. I also take a look at how the vegan movement can or should relate to the commercial world in general. After that, I examine some targets for institutional change, including policy, education, and organizations.

Improving the Alternatives

If people don't have good, valid alternatives for animal products, change becomes a lot harder. (Think again of the lack of alternatives for polluting airplanes.) I use the terms *improving* and *alternative* broadly. *Alternative* should be understood to cover not just products (food and otherwise) but services that don't entail animal suffering or exploitation. *Improving* applies not just to quality (mainly taste and texture, as well as healthfulness), but availability, variety, price, and other factors.

In providing alternatives, commercial companies complement the vegan movement and are a crucial ally. Most of what vegan advocates do is raise awareness and give people reasons and theories for not eating animal products, as well as practical tips to help them go vegan. But if we want people to apply this knowledge or put that awareness into practice, they'll need something to eat, and we need companies to produce that food.

Now, it goes without saying that veganism per se does not necessitate that we mimic omnivorism's commitment to processed foods; nor, for that matter, that the only food available is produced by commercial companies. A vegan diet can consist entirely of naturally occurring whole foods, which we can prepare with love for our friends and family each night. Indeed, some vegans argue that we need to move away from developing fancy cakes, cheese substitutes, or fake meats; or that we can make our own soymilk and tofu. I understand and honor this view. But I also live in the real world, where convenience and time are valuable commodities for harried commuters, busy parents, and professionals who eat only at restaurants or diners. Remember: Our task should be to make veganism *easier*.

Given that change often starts with behavior rather than attitude, the alternatives and the companies that make them become even more crucial. Apart from selling their products and offering alternatives, simply getting products into stores (with or without a VEGAN/VEGETARIAN/MEATFREE label) helps raise awareness about and mainstreams the idea that we can live without (or at least with fewer) animal products. Companies also have their own outreach channels: newsletters and social media through which they spread the vegan message, more or less explicitly. They can lobby to change laws on behalf of consumers, and they may at times sponsor or partner with organizations, projects, or initiatives in the vegan or animal advocacy movements.

New Kids on the Block

Vegetarian and vegan companies in many countries have spent decades of work developing and marketing meat and dairy alternatives. These enterprises can be large or small, local or multinational. Their products are sold in specialty food stores, but many also make it onto supermarket shelves. Recently, two new players have become involved: *disruptive start-ups* and *traditional meat companies.*

We've seen vegan startups for decades: from local stores to restaurants, from webshops to producers of alternatives. These ventures are a crucial part of the fledgling "vegeconomy," but they weren't usually established with the ambition of systemic change built into them. That factor distinguishes the disruptive startups, most of which originate in the US, especially California. These companies are looking to develop alternatives that could potentially topple entire sectors of the animal foods industry. Such game-changing ambitions require substantial investment, and these companies are usually funded with venture capital (VC). The solutions these companies arrive at are often hi-tech. Here are a few of them:

- Impossible Foods is developing the ideal plant-based burger (see box on p. 86).
- Beyond Meat does the same as Impossible Foods: their Beyond Chicken and Beyond Burger products are already in Whole Foods markets.
- New Wave Foods is trying to create synthetic shrimp from algae.
- Hampton Creek is working to take egg-laying hens out of the food chain by developing egg alternatives. Hampton has been successful at branding and marketing its Just Mayo vegan mayonnaise.
- Clara Foods has a similar mission as Hampton Creek, but is even more hi-tech. It's working on the world's first animal-free egg white, and is a division of IndieBio, the world's first synthetic biology accelerator, located in San Francisco.
- Perfect Day wants to produce a product that is chemically, nutritionally, and tastewise identical to milk, based on cow DNA but with otherwise no cow involved.
- Memphis Meats in Silicon Valley has already created the first meatball from cultured meat.
- In the Netherlands, the famous Vegetarian Butcher is a young company with the ambition of becoming the biggest "butcher" in

the world. In just a couple of years' time, the company is selling its products in four thousand outlets in fifteen countries. The Vegetarian Butcher works together with the world-famous agricultural university in Wageningen and the technical University in Delft to engineer and accelerate technological breakthroughs.

These startups hold some advantages compared to companies founded more than a decade ago, and their emergence has been facilitated by several new developments. Critical among these are new food technologies, a higher rate of awareness about the problems of animal agriculture (in which the vegan movement played an important part), and VC investment amounting to hundreds of millions of dollars over the last few years. These funds allow the entrepreneurs to recruit the best researchers, tech people, and marketers to develop and promote their products.

The investments also carry symbolic and signaling value. When famous VC firms such as Kleiner Perkins and Khosla Ventures, as well as change-makers such as Bill Gates, Google's Sergey Brin, or Li Ka-shing (the second-richest person in Asia) open their wallets, others take notice. The investors are signaling that animal products may have no or a very limited future. Readers who feel conflicted about capitalism may consider the possibility that these ventures are probably among the best things capitalism has to offer right now. Without the promise of earning money for their investors and shareholders, many of these companies wouldn't have been able to raise the necessary capital to establish their ambitious projects.

The second group of new players consists of traditional meat companies. More and more businesses that produce animal products are taking an interest in alternatives. One famous example is Rügenwalder Mühle, one of Germany's most respected and oldest meat companies, which has invested substantially in meat alternatives (see box on p. 90). Another is Tyson, the world's largest producer of chicken meat, which bought a five percent stake in Beyond Meat, and recently set up a $150 million fund to invest in startups, with the aim of investigating the possibilities of alternative protein.

It's not hard to see how some in the vegan movement might not be comfortable with such developments. It may irritate us when companies that make millions from killing animals are now trying to get their slice of the vegan pie or carve out a segment of the vegan cake, so to speak. Let's look at how the vegan movement can relate to companies, whether they exploit animals or not.

IMPOSSIBLE FOODS

Impossible Foods was founded by Patrick Brown, a professor emeritus at Stanford University widely acknowledged for his work in biochemistry. In 2009, Brown took a long sabbatical to think about what he wanted to do with his life. He decided to focus on one of the world's greatest environmental problems: animal agriculture. Brown founded Impossible Foods to develop a vegan alternative for meat, using his knowledge of biochemistry. He raised millions of dollars for his startup and even received (and declined) an offer from Google to acquire it. At the moment of going to press, the Impossible Foods burger is available at select locations in the US, and has just launched its first large-scale production facility. It has gotten ample media coverage, creating some hype for the burger. Its gimmick is that the heme-iron in it makes the burger appear to bleed when you fry it and put it on a plate. ∎

THE VEGAN MOVEMENT AND BUSINESS

The vegan movement's relationship to the corporate world is ambiguous, to say the least. Sometimes we lavish our love on a company for developing a new product or laud a restaurant for offering a new vegan dish. Sometimes we descend on their social media feeds like an angry mob when they offend us. Organizations, too, can work both positively and negatively, employing the carrot of communicating a company's good deeds or the stick of telling the entire vegan community (or the whole world) how evil that company is. Both methods are valid and can work, and this ambiguous relationship with companies is expected and understandable.

However, you can also find vegans who are profoundly skeptical or even cynical about the corporate world, and harbor anti-capitalist, anti-finance, and anti-commercial sentiments. These attitudes are mostly ideologically inspired and come from concerns about justice and equality, or from wariness about what they see as greed and a hunger for power.

Animal advocates have a choice whether to make trust or distrust our default attitude toward commerce. Although we should be on our guard, distrust as a default attitude can be unproductive and lead to many missed opportunities. That the first drive of any company is, by definition, continuity by profit is not in itself reason enough to distrust it. Fortunately, due in part to their visibility on social media, companies are paying more attention to accountability, sustainability, and an ethical approach to employment and their means of conducting commerce. At the same time, we as customers should keeping insisting on integrity, transparency, and corporate social responsibility in business.

The quest for profit is a powerful driver of change. At the moment, a lot of money is being poured into alternatives to animal products with the expectation that a lot of money will pour out—as well as a disruption of the entire social order. In such a circumstance, it's probably more strategic for vegan animal activists to make use of the profit motive rather than condemn and shun it. The reason why a commercial organization is presenting vegan products or services, starting to offer vegan dishes in restaurants, or selling them in a supermarket isn't all that important, even though it might make vegans feel better if a business is "in it for the animals." Whatever the entrepreneur and company's motivations, they are helping to change the system by shifting supply and demand, and (in case you find it important) you can take hope that companies themselves aren't immune to behaviors changing attitudes.

The fact that a company's first motive is profit means that it's not just the growth of the vegan-product category in general that matters, but the growth of the company's own brand. Thus, companies may compete with other businesses that sell vegan products. From a nonprofit perspective, this can appear strange. (I remember being initially confused by it when I had my first dealings with commercial enterprises.) But it's perfectly usual business practice.

BEING SPONSORED BY COMPANIES

From my time at EVA, the organization I founded, and from listening to people tell me about their experiences in other groups, I know that whether a nonprofit should or should not accept a certain business sponsorship can lead to complex and interminable internal debates. When the default sentiment toward the corporate world is distrust, many questions and caveats will need to be aired with the whole team or members and supporters. Questions will be asked about the company's integrity and whether associating with that business will damage or benefit the organization's reputation. There will be debates about whether the organization should make compromises or how much money it should ask for. Sometimes these collaborations—or even only discussions about them—will lead to schisms within the organization.

When you develop a good relationship with a company however, that business's sponsorship and support can be vital. When EVA was developing our Thursday Veggieday campaign, it was clear to us that the most obvious collaborator was a large producer of plant-based foods. We explained to the company how EVA's campaign emphasized the low environmental footprint and health aspects of plant-based foods, and how these arguments dovetailed with the values and objectives that the company wanted to have associated with its brand. We worked together for many years and the business's monetary sponsorship alone (in exchange for visibility in our campaign) was instrumental in making the campaign a success. ∎

Finally, I happen to believe that ambition and business acumen are attributes to be cherished, as is a healthy attention to the financial bottom line. Too many small vegan firms, made up of wonderful but impractical idealists, have failed. The animals need more than idealism and good intentions.

ALLY OR ENEMY?

Many companies can be potential allies, and vegan activists should work in tandem with them. Others can better be seen as the opposition. When vegans want to disrupt, it should be with the right (i.e., the *wrong*) companies and at the appropriate moments. My question is whether we can recognize allies when we see them.

Take the case of Tyson. One could wonder pragmatically whether Tyson is out to sabotage or slow down the vegan companies they invest in or believe idealistically that it's wrong for a commercial enterprise that makes money by killing animals to profit from the alternative. It's hard to be sure of either the motives of such businesses or the consequences of what they do, but here are some arguments for why I believe we should see them as allies.

First, behemoths like Tyson have a much greater potential to take a huge market share and reach many people that vegan companies or organizations can't. Think of Tyson's advertising budget alone for these products! Tyson possesses considerable financial and human capital, such as the R&D department, and their brand and retail franchises: their contracts with distributors, wholesalers, and retailers. It's important to realize that all these assets are "dual use" (for animal and non-animal products) and it's a reasonable supposition that the company is agnostic as to what ingredients go into their products, as long as there's a market and that market is profitable.

Secondly, the lobby *for* animal products is powerful. But as the industry's financial dependence on selling them decreases and its profits from vegan products increase, we can expect a shift from antagonism to support for vegan consumption. Plant-based milks may be an example of this. Some brands are now owned by enterprises that originally only sold dairy versions. Imagine how their opposition toward nondairy milks as an alternative may decrease once they have a stake in the nondairy category themselves. It's one of the reasons why Good Food Institute CEO Bruce Friedrich called the acquisition of Silk (an American soymilk producer) by Dean Foods (a traditional dairy behemoth) one of the best things that could have happened in the movement (Our Hen House).

HELPING COMPANIES HELP THE VEGAN MOVEMENT

If businesses can be influential and beneficial for the vegan movement, how can we help them help our cause? As individual customers, we can obviously choose which vendors or producers we patronize. We can talk

A MEAT COMPANY WITH AN IDENTITY CRISIS

Over the last few years, Rügenwalder Mühle, the ancient and deeply "respected" producer of all things meaty in Germany, has shifted its focus to vegetarian and vegan products, spending over €40 million on the promotion of meat alternatives, which is more than all other companies in Germany have spent *combined*. With the support and guidance of the Germany-based pro-vegan food awareness organization ProVeg International (formerly VEBU), Rügenwalder has reduced the number of eggs in their nonvegan products and introduced several more vegan products. Rügenwalder also supports the naming of meat alternatives the same as meat (i.e., vegan schnitzel can simply be called *schnitzel*)—a plan the farmers' union and even the Federal Ministry of Food, Agriculture, and Consumer Protection in Germany oppose. Rügenwalder is Example Number One of a meat company fighting for vegan issues while many of the traditional vegan companies themselves remain uninvolved in this kind of lobbying. The CEO of Rügenwalder has said that the company may not make meat from animals at all in twenty years and has called the meat-based sausage "the cigarette of the future." Ally or enemy? For me, the case is closed. ■

or write about companies or their products on blogs and social media and tell our friends about them. We can send these enterprises constructive feedback. Most particularly, we can avoid antagonizing them unnecessarily and recognize our allies when we see them. In most cases, I would argue, a boycott of vegan products because they're produced by an otherwise nonvegan company is counterproductive.

Unfortunately, vegans occasionally criticize people and businesses on our side of the fence. An example of unnecessary antagonism occurred with Daiya Foods, a Canadian company that for many vegans was the first to bring out a cheese that melted with all the gooeyness of dairy-based cheese. When the company displayed nonvegan recipes on its website, some vegans started a petition to boycott Daiya. Whereas an advocate wouldn't hand out leaflets in places where animal products were among the serving suggestions, expecting a company trying to reach mainstream consumers to do the same isn't realistic. As a minimum, vegans can simply choose to agree to disagree and let such an instance pass, instead of actively protesting against the firm.

On this point, legendary animal activist Henry Spira (talking about alternatives for animal tests) has advice that I believe vegans should heed in all such cases:

> If people are going to develop alternatives, it's the people in the research community who will be developing alternatives. If you're going to get the regulatory agencies to change their requirements, it's going to be animal researchers who are the ones who are going to do it, it's not going to be us who are going to do it. I mean, these are the folks that you need if you're going to be serious about change. . . . You're not going to reprogram them by saying we're saints and you're sinners, and we're going to clobber you with a two-by-four in order to educate you. (Singer 1998, p. 113)

The Daiya boycott probably had a great deal to do with vegans' expectations. We don't anticipate much vegan-product generation or market outreach from a giant meat company. Therefore, when a business we thought was vegan "slips up" and disappoints us, we're irritated. Such annoyance is a profoundly human reaction, but it makes little sense and it's generally unproductive.

If we animal advocates want be more concrete in our support of companies, we should look to our own organizations. Most obviously, this would be by helping to increase demand for those goods or services. When, thanks in part to our outreach (and factors outside of our control), demand for vegan food increases, the pie gets bigger and the companies selling vegan products have more to split among them. Vegan or animal advocacy organizations can raise general awareness, or highlight specific companies, brands, or products in their outreach. The latter can be part of a formal sponsorship collaboration, or simply because the organization likes the company or products and thinks more people (both omnivores and vegans) should know about either. We can publish product or restaurant reviews, thus sending more

PLANTBASED SOLUTIONS

Animal advocates can start a company to help other businesses, vegan or not. David Benzaquen worked in fundraising and advocacy for various animal protection groups, such as Farm Sanctuary before founding a company called PlantBased Solutions in 2012. Its aim is to help market vegan consumer products to the world. David and his team manage a number of areas for their clients, including marketing, branding, fundraising, and more. His clients have included Gardein, Green Monday, Miyoko's Kitchen, and Treeline Cheese. David believes that although education and advocacy are vital tools to raise awareness, the animal advocacy movement should also focus more on using the market to advance vegan living. He feels that by taking on this previously unaddressed strategy, he's making a greater difference than when he was replicating the same activist strategies as his peers in the nonprofit sector. ■

people to the company. We can place paid advertising in our magazines or on our websites. Or we can even present awards to the best products to garner public attention.

Larger or more established vegan and animal advocacy organizations may possess in-house expertise that offers businesses consultations that may prove valuable to them. They may be able to help companies extend their range, correct flaws or mistakes in products or packaging, train chefs and buyers, and help in other ways. They can endorse products and present unique insights into the market of "heavy users," and provide channels to reach them.

ProVeg International has a whole startup department. It offers seminars, videos, and individual coaching for vegan entrepreneurs and has supported hundreds of vegans who wish to open their own businesses. They even provide loans. ProVeg also has its own testing community to help new and more established companies test-market their products and receive feedback.

Another practice through which vegan organizations can help businesses is by informing and educating their own supporters (sympathizers, donors, members, subscribers). Organizations can help supporters open their minds to the possibility that not all meat companies are necessarily enemies. They can encourage them to get over their suspicions about money and investors, and to appreciate the benefits of science and technology. Given the interest of many vegans in natural or organic foods, many of them may be even more distrustful of food they perceive as "unnatural" or processed, or dependent on technology than the general population.

Clean meat offers a case in point. *Clean meat* is flesh developed from animal cells without slaughtering the animals involved. There are good reasons to be excited about the potential of clean meat. It could be the technological revolution that precedes a moral transformation. The prospects for product growth are good. Researchers are confident that in the next five or ten years they'll be able to overcome most technological barriers. Furthermore, the price of the product should eventually drop enough to make it competitive with conventional meat.

Clean meat can be more sustainable (requiring less energy, water, or fertilizer), healthier (it's easy to control the fat content, for example) and safer (a lower risk of all kinds of contamination and the danger to workers from the slaughtering process) than conventional meat. Beyond the technological and regulatory challenges facing clean meat is public perception. The production of clean meat is obviously more hi-tech and seems less "natural" than what we're used to. "Natural," however, is a confusing and not particularly useful concept here. Not only are the animals who are trucked to the slaughterhouse full of chemicals and hormones, but they are killed and dismembered using a wide array of electrical and mechanical tools. Where is the inherent "naturalness" of this process? Furthermore, we might add, not everything natural is good for us (namely radioactivity) and not everything human-made is negative (penicillin is a case in point).

Genetically modified organisms (GMOs) are another example of a natural/unnatural confusion. Many people, including vegans, are opposed to their use. In certain circles, it's almost taboo to say that you're ambivalent or agnostic about even researching their potential. In theory at least, GMO products could reduce animal testing and create better alternatives, as well as grow plants with higher nutrient profiles, increased agricultural yield, and requiring fewer pesticides.[11] Although it's necessary to be careful with new technologies, it's important to retain some objectivity and not judge them on the basis of hearsay, emotions, or ideology. The American startup Clara Foods is developing a substitute for egg whites. The substitute, however, is based on genetically modified yeast, which means that many companies and consumers might be wary of adopting it. Currently, it wouldn't be allowed in the European Union.

In the case of clean meat and GMOs, vegans should distinguish between principled objections (e.g., on the naturalness of genetic modification) and practical or situational objections (e.g., a concern for monopolies or the privatization of public knowledge and resources).

Consumers in the vegan movement can be innovators or early adopters of new food products and technologies. If we want these to succeed, we should lend our support, while of course never letting down our guard.

When Vegans Mean Business

People who want to earn a living by making the world a better place often end up in a nonprofit organization, if they're lucky. That path seems the most obvious one for changemakers. However, entering or starting a business can offer several advantages over nonprofits. A company has an easier time making money and can be more sustainable than an organization that has to scrape together its funds from donors and/or subsidies every year. Businesses can also be more scalable and thus potentially have a wider reach or more influence. Some advantages of nonprofits are that they can work with volunteers, can receive subsidies and donations, and can often count on more goodwill and enthusiasm than a company can. One aspect that can go both ways is credibility. At first sight, nonprofits may look trustworthier because they don't appear to be

Islands and Infiltrators

Vegan restaurants and shops are examples of what I call *islands* amid a sea of omnivorous establishments. *Infiltrators*, on the other hand, are vegan products in supermarkets, or vegan dishes on the menu of a regular restaurant. When we vegans are influencing influencers and changing institutions, we're usually attempting to insert infiltrators.

Islands make vegans feel good. We don't need to walk past shelves or counters of animal products, and we don't need to worry about meat or dairy in our dishes or on our plates. We may feel ethically more comfortable by spending our money on islands. Nonetheless, infiltrators are crucial if we want to reach new customers and get more exposure among omnivores, many of whom will never enter a vegan restaurant or specialty shop, and will never buy a vegan cookbook. One problem in today's market is that vegan stuff is seen as stuff for vegans, and omnivores will pass over the vegan option because they're not vegan, just as the non-diabetic among us might avoid a dish labeled "suitable for diabetics." ∎

motivated by money. But they *also* have an agenda. (Animal rights organizations are not the most reliable sources of health information, it may be thought.) Moreover, to business folks, nonprofits may not always be the most dependable partners.

The borders between for-profit and nonprofit structures are less clear-cut than they used to be. Many nonprofits look to earn income, whereas companies can have corporate social responsibility or volunteer programs. In between are social enterprises, wherein the social objective is the raison d'être of the business. Rather than maintaining the old profit-versus-nonprofit dichotomy, it may be more useful for activists to consider a spectrum of engagement, ranging from "finance first" to "impact first," with many hybrid possibilities in between.

Some of the disruptive startups I mentioned above are strange beasts. The entrepreneurs in question seem to have founded them with the goal of helping to solve the environmental, ethical, or health problems inherent in animal products, and so appear more like social enterprises. That perception is what allows a company like Memphis Meats, which wants to make slaughtered-animal meat history by replacing it with clean meat, to set up a crowdfunding campaign to raise money from its supporters. That said, most of these businesses have received venture capital, and we can safely assume that investors will want a profit from their investment. Hence, in spite of the noble aim of changing the world, such companies have to make a profit, which, as we saw, isn't necessarily at the expense of promoting veganism or changing social realities.

Of course, apart from founding a multimillion-dollar enterprise that tries to disrupt the whole meat industry, you can also start your own small or medium-sized concern, such as a restaurant, store, or local company. You can even monetize more direct forms of advocacy, making a living from your blog, website, podcast, or YouTube channel.

OTHER TARGETS FOR CREATING A FACILITATING ENVIRONMENT

So far in this chapter we've concentrated on companies producing and offering vegan products. But we can influence many other institutions

Helping Chickens: Karen Davis and Josh Tetrick

To illustrate two radically different approaches to helping animals, let's look at two completely different people.

Karen Davis, founder and director of United Poultry Concerns (UPC), has committed much of her life to raising awareness about and advocating for one of the most maligned animals on the planet: chickens (as well as other poultry). Karen runs a chicken haven in Virginia and UPC does educational outreach about chickens and the suffering that's involved in the production of their meat and eggs.

Josh Tetrick, founder of Hampton Creek, wants to help chickens by creating alternatives for eggs. In the US, Just Mayo is the only Hampton Creek brand used by the Compass Group, the world's largest catering company, and by all 7-Eleven stores for the preparation of their sandwiches. Just Mayo is also available at Walmart, Target, Costco, and other giant retailers. That's a huge number of chickens' eggs that are *not* being laid or consumed.

I juxtapose UPC and Hampton Creek not just to highlight a nonprofit versus a for-profit career, but to show how we can have the same objective by campaigning for moral awareness *and* through a tweaking of the environment by providing alternatives. ■

to create a facilitating environment. These are any commercial business, governmental institution, major NGO, educational establishment, hospital, or insurance company, to name a few. All can be influencers or multipliers. They can broadcast our message to many more people than we can reach by ourselves. They may be large structures with thousands of employees, many of whom eat every day in the canteen. They can also be influential beyond their own structure, such as with an organization that provides programs on or advocates for health or sustainability.

Institutions obviously vary in their reach, but you can almost always be more effective by approaching individuals who represent those institutions than by talking to individuals in the street. You could lobby environmental and health NGOs to incorporate messages about the sustainability or health implications of meat consumption in their campaigning. ProVeg International successfully lobbied large environmental groups such as Greenpeace, WWF, and Friends of the Earth to include a 50 percent reduction of livestock in Germany as one of its carbon-emissions objectives. The joint position paper of the so-called climate alliance in Germany lists this precise goal.

You could contact an association of doctors or dieticians to educate their members about talking to their patients regarding animal products. You could meet with local, statewide, or national political figures responsible for meals in the school system. Or you could encourage a large company, serving meals to thousands of employees, to introduce more vegan options in their cafeteria.

INFLUENCING THE INFLUENCERS

ProVeg International has made influencing the influencers their core focus. ProVeg persuaded one of the largest and most respected hospital and medical research facilities in Europe to set up a conference on the health aspects of vegan diets. The 2016 gathering attracted over a thousand people, most of whom were medical professionals or medical students. ProVeg worked with the Compass Group in Germany to train and inspire the company to offer more plant-based meals. According to ProVeg's founder Sebastian Joy, influencers must speak the language of those they wish to influence. They should know what they want and frame their argument as something that's in the best interests of the person they want to sway. Joy also states that ProVeg's strategic positioning as a pro-veg-food organization rather than an animal rights organization gives them more credibility and a better reputation to work with a variety of influencers, such as health institutions, caterers, the media, and meat companies. ∎

CHANGE IN EDUCATION

Schools are a critical area for institutional change. Schools can reach many pupils, who may not only be consumers, voters, and citizens, but who also may get inspired to choose a career path in which they contribute further to developing or spreading plant-based solutions. That's why an organization like the Good Food Institute invests significantly in presentations at top universities in the US that traditionally have educated many future social-change agents and business movers and shakers.

Another good example of successful institutional change within an educational context is the efforts of the Humane Society of the United States (HSUS) to help more than two hundred school districts, over a hundred universities, and sixty hospitals in the United States to adopt programs like Meatless Monday. Among those districts are those of Los Angeles, Houston, Dallas, and San Diego, good for a total of over one million meals served every day. HSUS has also worked with the biggest caterers and partnered with the US military to try to reduce meat consumption at its military bases. On another continent, the Brazilian Vegetarian Society has been instrumental in introducing the Meatless Monday program in São Paulo (actually on Tuesdays), providing about one million meals on meatless days.

Within the field of education, special attention should go to training chefs. Almost all chefs at any level are trained to cook meat dishes, and by the time they graduate have little to no experience or knowledge of vegan cooking. HSUS has developed a two-day plant-based culinary intensive course and trained almost eight hundred chefs in 2016. With the support of the EU, vegetarian and vegan organizations in Austria, Belgium, Germany, and the Netherlands developed "Vegucation," a program in which chefs and chef trainers are provided with vegan-cooking classes. Organizations in different countries have also staged vegan contests for chefs, which may help to lift the image of plant-based cooking to another level.

It goes without saying that outreach in schools can also focus on advocacy rather than changing meals or developing cooking skills. In

Israel, the organization Anonymous for Animals is reaching over 25,000 students a year by means of lectures given by a small army of volunteers.

LEGAL CHANGE

Sometimes institutions, and companies especially, can adopt pro-vegan or pro-animal measures voluntarily, with or without the instigation of an animal or vegan organization. Wonderful though this may be, there's no guarantee the change will survive the next president or CEO, a drop in profit, or backlash from employees or customers. Moreover, whereas one or a few companies may take these steps, a majority of others may not yet get onboard. Ultimately then, legislative action offers the best although not absolute guarantee of institutional change. A case in point is that, a few decades ago, some restaurants and bars declared themselves smoke-free. Today, in many countries they're all legally obliged to be smoke-free. The difference in compliance and repercussions is enormous.

There are many legal changes we could strive to get on the legislative agenda. Most obviously are laws that reform the uses of animals: to increase the welfare (even if minimally) for animals raised for food or used in research or entertainment. These would include larger cages, reducing the distance the animals are transported to slaughter, and other improvements. But legal changes could involve different facets of food production. In Portugal, a recently approved law stipulates that all public canteens must provide vegan meals. This came about as a result of the Portuguese Vegetarian Society collecting over 15,000 signatures to petition for this provision. Similarly, the organization Sentience Politics in Switzerland has launched several ballot initiatives to demand plant-based options in public canteens in various Swiss cities. The International Vegan Rights Alliance and ProVeg International have planned the international legal symposium on veganism and law, which covers many of the legal aspects of promoting a vegan diet.

Vegan organizations also could help lobby for laws to make things easier for producers of vegan items, such as ensuring that in Europe cow and plant-based milks carry the same sales tax. One obvious, although controversial, legal change would be a health or CO_2 tax on meat and other animal products. The animal-products industry can obviously lobby to change laws in its favor or keep others off the books; it certainly has the money to do it. That power is why it's doubly important for the animal advocacy movement to raise funds to compete and form coalitions.

The Eurogroup of Animals, for example, is a pan-European association of animal welfare organizations. Together, they lobby EU institutions to deliver better animal welfare legislation and enforcement. Cooperation like this recently emerged in the business field, among plant-based stakeholders. The Plant-based Food Association in the US is a group of dozens of companies selling vegan products or services, which together lobby for their interests (and thus their customers' interests) with lawmakers. In the Netherlands, the Green Protein Alliance has a similar aim.

Choice Architecture

I have already touched on how people don't like to be persuaded and don't always like moral arguments to be thrown at them, as they can feel judged or guilty (more about this in chapter 5). An overreliance on moral arguments can be even more awkward when we're demanding institutional change. Decision-makers are pragmatic. They need to be shown that their actions will have a concrete result and that you'll deliver support. Their eyes rarely well up with tears when advocates describe animal suffering. They're usually wary of telling people what to do and don't see it as their place to meddle with people's choices about what they eat.

The positive outcome of what I've discussed in this chapter is that advocates don't need moral arguments in all situations. We can tweak people's environment so they do the right thing without knowing it. You may have heard about how supermarkets place premium products at eye level on the shelves so the customer's attention and money will be directed to them more easily. This technique can also be used for doing good. School or company cafeterias have experimented with putting healthy options in more easily accessible places, such as water placed more prominently than soft drinks.

LOBBYING FOR ANIMAL RIGHTS

One of the key components of animal advocacy is legal rights for animals. In the first chapter I described how dependent we are on the use of animals. In such a situation, it will be almost impossible to give basic legal rights to animals, particularly those we use for food. A law that granted an animal raised for food some degree of personhood would naturally lead to no more consumption of meat and dairy products.

At the moment, most people may give lip service to the notion of animal rights but their actions toward animals used for food suggest otherwise. This reality doesn't mean that we shouldn't continue to advocate for the rights of farmed animals, but we need to be aware that this highly ambitious demand may alienate a lot of people, including those in decision-making positions. It's my belief that when our dependency on the use of animals diminishes, it will be much easier to establish rights for pigs and chickens and cows.

Until then, it makes most sense to campaign for the rights of individuals of certain species—such as lions, pandas, and elephants—whose relationship with us is less instrumental, and to insist on a greater consistency of rights toward members of the same species, such as a beagle who is a companion in our home but an experimental subject in a laboratory.

Primates, for example, belong to the same species as we do. In recent years, the use and abuse of these relatives has come under increasing social, legislative, and legal scrutiny. The Great Ape Project aims to defend the rights of nonhuman great apes, based (among other arguments) on the fact that we're genetically similar to them (chimpanzees and humans can donate blood to one another). The Nonhuman Rights Project, led by legal scholar Steven Wise, is advocating for chimpanzees to be accorded the right not to be imprisoned against their will, based upon the notion that legal persons can sue for a writ of habeas corpus. Asking for rights for cetaceans offers another realistic option, because many people recognize their intelligence and uniqueness, or simply are fond of them, and because in most countries people aren't dependent on using them. Establishing rights for these animals could blaze the trail for the rights of other animals in the future. ■

This is called "choice architecture" or "nudging." People receive a gentle push in the right direction and so make good choices without knowing it (Thaler and Sunstein). As long as they don't notice or don't care about the "tweak," people's persuasion-resistance isn't triggered (Knowles and Linn). They don't feel they're being sold something and keep thinking of themselves as autonomous individuals who can make their own decisions.

One promising feature of choice architecture is to change the default option, which is the choice or action made without any effort. In most countries, for example, the default is that your organs will *not* be available for the critically ill after you die. Countries that have reversed the default option obviously have many more organ donors. An example from our domain might be the meal on a long-distance flight. At the moment, you have to make an effort and a special request if you want the vegan option. Imagine if the default meal for all passengers were vegan! I've always wondered why it wasn't anyway, given the many different nationalities, religions, and allergic passengers onboard the plane and how such would cut the total CO_2 emissions of the plane as well as reduce the potential for sickness due to inadequate meat preparation. In the flipped scenario, those omnivores who complained would be told by the flight attendant that they should have ordered the meat option in advance.

EVA has operationalized a "nudge" in collaboration with city schools in Ghent, Belgium. On Thursday (the Veggieday), the default school lunch is vegetarian, with the result that 94 percent of children eat vegetarian food on Thursday. Choice architecture provided a terrific means to contribute without preaching. Beyond the direct effect, interventions like these can normalize plant-based food for the long run. Furthermore, this strategy avoids people feeling their freedom of choice is being taken away. Children can still have meat-based meals, but they need to make an effort. EVA made the good thing the easy thing, at least on Thursdays.

THE IMPORTANCE OF PROFESSIONAL ORGANIZATIONS

The larger the influence of a company, organization, or politician, the more rewarding and challenging it is to lobby them. It's hard to change laws whatever your cause, and politicians responsible for drafting or voting for new legislation will either need to feel they have enough of the public behind them or be highly skilled, motivated, and courageous.

In most cases, our push for institutional, including legal, change will require professional organizations rather than grassroots groups or individual effort. Professional organizations often represent sizable constituencies, and some institutions, especially political ones, will only be moved to action if they see that the association speaks for or can influence a significant number of people. Organizations often have resources that individual activists or smaller groups don't always possess, and thus are able to conduct research, show certain results to institutional partners, and reach out to tens of thousands or even millions of followers. They can leverage their channels to put pressure on the other party—to make them stop or urge them on. They also have more money, which is useful for setting up campaigns, lobbying, attracting professional talent, and other benefits that money can buy.

The extra expertise of organizations may be necessary to educate the institution on different topics and show why the cause is socially relevant. Such expertise needs to be skilled in diplomacy, lobbying, and politics. Another advantage an organization has is that, as a well-established structure, it can more easily guarantee the continuity of the actions and campaigns. Individual and grassroots initiatives may in that sense be much more fragile.

Some vegans, especially individuals who are unaffiliated with groups, are critical of large organizations. They blame them for making compromises and "selling out." They accuse them of raising money simply to maintain their existence or of sleeping with the enemy. Anyone who's ever worked with an institution will know that change requires pragmatism and compromise. Institutional partners or allies usually won't do exactly what animal rights or vegan groups suggest. They'll not necessarily spread the precise message we want. They may not share our ideology and they may believe their own constituency isn't ready for our demands or message. For example, in my experience, when institutional partners want to conduct outreach about plant-based food among their audience, they feel more comfortable emphasizing the health and environmental consequences of eating animals than whether it is ethically sound.

When others don't agree completely with what we vegans want, we have a choice. If we're too idealistic, we may find it hard or impossible to associate ourselves with nonvegan restaurants, accept sponsorship from or advertising from businesses that sell vegan *and* nonvegan products, work with schools that put vegan *and* omnivorous dishes on the menu, collaborate with groups that still support non–animal friendly causes, associate with TV chefs who usually cook with animal recipes . . . and the litany continues. With parties that don't share *all* our ideals, collaboration can be complicated. So one option is to refuse to work with them. That way we will avoid "contamination" from whatever they're doing and not receive criticism from other vegans.

Our other option is to be pragmatic: we compromise and accept the imperfect manner in which our partners will bring the message to their voters, members, customers, or employees. When deciding whether to collaborate or not, our decision will depend on the perceived gains and the perceived sacrifices. If we don't want to be pragmatic, we'll have many fewer chances of starting alliances that may help influence significant numbers of people. If we don't compromise, we may end up working and preaching on an island.

Vegan activist Matt Ball puts it like this:

Many groups have condemned themselves to acrimonious anonymity and burnout. They cut themselves off from consideration by the public, and do not provide any incentive for change within the animal industries. More diverse organizations, on the other hand, have attracted broad memberships of vegetarians and non-vegetarians. They achieve results because they can reach out to individuals and business that may not share all of their opinions. (Ball, p. 106)

A Word on Money

To change the environment and influence multipliers, to acquire skills from experts, to increase the depth and width of outreach channels, and to spread information—organizations need money. Although organizations are sometimes criticized for how much time and how many resources they invest in raising funds, the emphasis on donations is entirely natural and necessary. Of course, one hopes that organizations are transparent on where or from whom they get their money and how they spend it. As members or supporters we should hold them accountable. Organizations are not immune to stupid choices, poor strategy, bad management, and extravagant wages for certain functions. These are the risks of professionalism in any movement, and not just among vegans or animal advocates.

It's also true that, intentional misconduct aside, organizations may become less dynamic and raise funds simply to keep staff. Organizations need to be aware of this risk, and can use their members and donors to help them guard against it. However, whereas corruption and inefficiency should be called out, fundraising shouldn't. There's no shame in seeking donations, recruiting members, or having a large budget. And it's entirely normal that in most organizations the most significant part of the budget is staff salaries.

It's a fascinating aspect of human attitudes toward social change that so many of us are suspicious of money in the nonprofit sector. We seem to have no problem with people earning a substantial salary from selling laundry detergents or making video games, but we're highly critical when those working for the public good are allowed to lead a comfortable life. Isn't it unfortunate that it's so difficult to earn a living by doing good? Many of us would love to work fulltime for animals or some other worthy cause, but we can't because there aren't enough paid jobs available at anything like a livable wage. The more successful fundraisers are at their work, and the more entrepreneurial individual activists can become, the better this must be for advocates, organizations, the vegan movement, and the animals we care about so much.

Animal Rights or Vegan Organizations?

If we need substantial, professional organizations, we should also ask: What kind? In our movement, we have two of them. Animal rights organizations primarily or exclusively talk about animal rights, while vegan ones (the typical vegan societies or groups in many countries) use all arguments, even though the motivation of workers or volunteers for these groups will be mostly a concern for animals, too. Because, as we've suggested, people can start out on their path to Veganville due to health or sustainability concerns and then adopt a care for animals, it makes sense to include organizations in the animal advocacy and vegan movements that don't emphasize the ethical argument more than other arguments.

Generally speaking, most major organizations in the movement are animal rights–oriented. With some exceptions, they're larger, more active, and more dynamic than most vegan groups. This reality might be because it's harder to raise money and grow membership for veganism, which doesn't necessarily hold the emotional appeal of animal suffering. Animal rights groups can advocate for issues beyond agriculture (such as companion animals, fur, and animals in entertainment or research), which is unusual for vegan organizations. The latter rarely campaign for animal-welfare issues, which can be a great tool to recruit supporters and donors. Animal rights organizations find it easier to recruit committed volunteers. Ending cruelty to animals is a strong motivator, and protesting animal abuse or participating in direct action is to many, especially young, people more attractive than describing the negative effects on the environment or building campaigns around other topics.

Yet, vegan organizations have some advantages. They can more easily attract people who aren't interested in animals, but are worried about climate change, pollution, world hunger, or their health. Vegan groups often emphasize food, taste, and lifestyle. All these reasons (and others that are less important) are different roads by which to reach Veganville. Animal rights organizations can include these other factors in their outreach, too, but they may sound less credible than when used by a vegan organization and obviously much less credible than when used by a health or environmental organization.

The animal argument is the only one to reduce consumption to zero. But it's *at present* less credible and less relevant socially and politically. Animals, whether we vegan activists like it or not, also constitute a more controversial, sensitive, and dangerous topic than the others. Witness the resistance against it in the US, where several animal rights activities have fallen under antiterrorism legislation.

The takeaway from my observations above is that, given the present landscape in the animal advocacy movement, we don't have enough large, vibrant vegan (non-animal rights) organizations that can successfully do the following things, among others:

- Lobby governments on the sustainability and health problems surrounding animal products
- Lobby health and environmental organizations to focus on the problem of animal products
- Work with producers, restaurants, and other businesses to improve and extend their vegan offerings
- Work with chefs, cooking schools, and educational establishments to raise the bar for vegan cooking and improve training

The table opposite gives an overview of differences between animal rights and vegan organizations:

	ANIMAL RIGHTS ORGANIZATIONS	VEGAN ORGANIZATIONS
Internal motivation	Animals	
Arguments used	Exclusively or mainly animals	Animals, environment, health, global hunger
Welfare reforms	Campaigned for, ignored, or against	Not campaigned for
Other animals than farmed animals	Often campaigned for	Not campaigned for or get only little attention
Examples of bigger orgs (paid staff of ten or more) that more or less fit in here	Mercy for Animals, Animal Equality, Humane League, Compassion over Killing, Vegan Outreach, PETA, Djurensrätt (Sweden), HSUS, CIWF, Animals Australia, SAFE (New Zealand), Anonymous (Israel)	ProVeg International, Vegan Society (UK), EVA, Good Food Institute
Advantages	• More emotional appeal • Easier to fundraise • Can talk about other animal issues than food as gate openers • Easier to recruit committed staff and volunteers • Easier to wage welfare campaigns	• More credibility with policy makers • Easier to get subsidies • Easier to collaborate with many stakeholders on different topics
Disadvantages	• Less credibility on topics other than animals • More controversial	• Harder to get large number of members • Harder to fundraise

CONCLUSION

Creating a facilitating environment is a means of bypassing the need for an individual to be highly motivated. By tweaking the environment—developing better products and rearranging local cafeterias, educating chefs, influencing prices, and lobbying for new laws—it's possible to make it easy to do good.

The playing field for social change has varied greatly over the years. Now, more than ever, companies are important drivers of change. In trying to influence the corporate world—from producers to retailers—the vegan animal advocacy movement must use both carrot and stick. We can pressure companies to force them to change direction and adopt more animal-friendly or veg-friendly practices. But we must also help producers research, develop, and market vegan products, even if the company in question does the same with animal products.

Institutional, business, structural, political outreach—and contacting influencers and multipliers—require solid organizations within the vegan animal advocacy movement that are well-funded so they can attract the necessary talent and expertise. Some of the most promising organizations today may be groups like the Good Food Institute, which approaches institutions with a non-moral and pragmatic message (see opposite). 🌍

THE GOOD FOOD INSTITUTE AND OTHERS

The last few years have seen the emergence of innovative organizations that focus on food but largely avoid animal advocacy in their communication, even though concern for animals lies at the heart of their foundation. One of them is the Good Food Institute (GFI), created by Mercy for Animals but now operating independently. GFI promotes and develops competitive alternatives to meat, dairy, and eggs. To do that, GFI works with a chain of stakeholders, from scientists, entrepreneurs, and investors to distributors and retailers. GFI is especially hopeful about clean-meat technologies and educates institutions about plant-based and clean-meat research and development. GFI's professional mission, communication, and appearance make it a particularly credible partner for the stakeholders it wants to collaborate with or lobby.

Two other recently founded nonprofits are New Harvest, which aims to accelerate breakthroughs in cellular agriculture, and the Modern Agriculture Foundation, a completely volunteer-based group that focuses on developing clean chicken–meat.

In Australia, Thomas King, a young activist, realized there was an enormous opportunity to help animals, the planet, and human health by launching a credible body focused on promoting innovative meat alternatives in the region. He left his position in animal advocacy to start a new organization called Food Frontier. This organization, too, will focus on institutional change and emphasize health and environmental aspects more than moral ones.

Note that just as these organizations don't emphasize the moral aspects of eating animal products, so they also omit the word *vegan* from the name of their organization, for strategic reasons. ∎

5

Support

Encouraging Every Step

"Communication is what the listener does."—**Peter Drucker**

We've focused on the call to action, the arguments, and the environment. Now, we look at our roles as supporters and catalysts. We want to communicate with people so that as many as possible start, continue, and finish the trek to Veganville. To do this, we'll need to encourage them, give directions, and tell them when and where to take a break. We can talk in a manner that makes them more likely to start or continue, *or* discourages them. Most importantly, we also need to *listen* to them. In short, this chapter is about communicating with our audience, whether as an individual or as a group, whether one-to-one or as a broadcast, whether to a passerby in the street or an influential person like the CEO of a catering company. One principle will be central: When we communicate, we should put ourselves in our audience's shoes.

An important part of our task is to welcome others to our group. To that end, in this chapter I also take a pragmatic look at the concept of veganism. Most of this book has been about reduction. I've emphasized, however, that this should be complementary to a vegan message, so it's time to examine how we'd frame that message.

When reading this chapter, keep in mind the main points from what we've learned so far:

- A large group of meat reducers may be a better way to change the system as they drive demand and supply. Becoming stricter gets easier as there are more options and social acceptance grows.

- We don't need to use moral arguments all the time. Non-moral motivations can develop into moral ones, and compassion can grow after people have taken the first steps, for whatever reasons.
- We have to create a facilitating environment by working on institutional change.

AUDIENCE-CENTERED COMMUNICATION

"You never really understand a person until you consider things from his point of view."—**Harper Lee**

A LICENSE TO INFLUENCE

As I have explained, it's not just the vegan movement that creates change for animals: businesses, health and environmental organizations, and all sorts of institutions may do so more indirectly, with or without vegans influencing them. Nevertheless, the vegan movement will continue to play an important role for the foreseeable future. The strength of our movement lies in the skillsets of our members or adherents. The more effectively and eloquently we communicate and advocate, the more progress we'll make.

I'm talking about *communication* here in a particularly broad sense. It's not just how we speak or write but everything others might see and experience relating to us. *Communication* is what we post on social media, our behavior in restaurants, how we cook, what we eat, how we shop. It's what we read, what we watch, what we share. It's the clothes we wear and how we look. It's our general attitude, especially in certain circumstances. (Are we cheerful or miserable?) It's everything.

Some people are more effective advocates for animals than others. Some of us may be too loud, others too quiet. The former may be *too* assured of their beliefs and have developed a style of advocacy that can push beyond effectiveness. The latter may be too shy or believe they have no business talking to others about what they should eat. We need to strike a balance in our outreach between these extremes.

As for the quiet ones: If our desire to change things is based on both rational arguments and empathy, it's perfectly acceptable to try to influence people. Obviously, we shouldn't try to *force* people to adopt our vegan diet—in fact, much of this book is exactly about how *not* to do that—but I want to stress that we shouldn't be ashamed or embarrassed about wanting to open people's hearts and minds. There's nothing special about advocacy. Everyone making a sale, every mom or dad, every child, every husband or wife tries to change someone else's mind—often for much-less-noble objectives than ours. Furthermore, even if we don't want to, we can't help influencing people around us.

It should be said that no friend of animals should believe they don't have the right to influence others when they're not vegan or even vegetarian. *Anyone* can do good for animals. We shouldn't think that a nonvegan can do nothing right, whereas a vegan can do nothing wrong. We shouldn't consider nonvegan animal advocacy less valuable than the mere fact of being a vegan (even a non-active one). It should be beyond any doubt that people like Jonathan Safran Foer, with his book *Eating Animals*, or the philosopher Peter Singer (author of *Animal Liberation*) were more consequential in reducing animal consumption than almost any one of us could ever dream of, and neither of them is (strictly) vegan.

A MATTER OF CHOICE?

People may tell us that what they eat is a matter of choice ("I respect vegans," they'll add). We should, of course, respect people's freedom to choose, but at the same time we can make clear, when appropriate, that they're not talking about picking the color for the new wallpaper in their living room. For the animals it's not a question of blue or green, but suffering or not suffering, a matter of life and death. Although everyone is *still* free to choose what to eat, we can at least say that those who choose vegetarian or vegan food have more solid arguments for their choice than omnivores have for theirs. Everyone who cares about rational conversation should take that into account.

Moreover, it's not as if the general population is choosing freely what to eat. People are influenced by what supermarkets, producers, and restaurants coax them to eat. Subsidies and governmental policies skew the market to make some foods more available and cheaper than others. We're all affected by prices and promotions. It's hard to choose what's on our plates independently of what our parents, grandparents, or other people in our nation or culture eat or ate. Most of us are only under the *illusion* that we're free to eat what we want. We're all affected by the belief system that Melanie Joy calls carnism (2010). Our vegan voice won't limit our omnivorous friends any further; it might even liberate them.

We should consider our influence no different from that of the media, family, or peers. We should, however, avoid being coercive or manipulative. Trying to influence another person is not a crime, but it *is* an art. It starts with not thinking in terms of *persuading* people, but rather in helping them to open up; not behaving like a moral crusader, judge, or police officer, but as a supporter. ■

OUR OBJECTIVE: IMPACT

When communicating (again, broadly conceived), it's vital always to bear one question in mind: *Am I making a real impact for the animals?* You may think: *Of course, what else?* But let's look at some of the other motivations we may consciously or unconsciously be paying too much attention to.

Impact is not about speaking our truth. If we're asked at dinner why we're vegan and we launch into the gruesome suffering of animals, we may be speaking the truth—and *our* truth—but we may be alienating some people at the table. In this case, conveying our truth is not that important, and can be counterproductive. The more subjective the truth we're discussing, the more problematic it can be. Statements such as "meat is murder" or "dairy is rape" are subject to interpretation (see box on the next page). We're not betraying ourselves or the animals when we don't speak those kinds of truth. On the contrary, we're doing the animals the greatest favor when we think about what changes people.

Impact is not about being right. Whether we're talking about our *belief* that we're objectively right, or we actually *are* objectively right, being correct or consistent doesn't necessarily have any genuine effect on what we want to achieve. We may by definition be accurate in arguing that eating animals is murder, but if another person doesn't agree, it's moot. We all love to be right (It's a great feeling!), so we often pursue this goal over anything else. But if we're constantly seeking a self-righteous rush, we may miss learning something because we don't want our interlocutor to show us contradictory (yet perhaps equally correct and true) arguments.

Impact is not about winning an argument. Even if the other person tells us we're right, we haven't necessarily had a positive effect. A saying from sales is "win an argument, lose a customer." When the other person feels they've lost, they may feel even less sympathetic toward us or our cause. Benjamin Franklin says: "If you argue and rankle and contradict, you may achieve a victory sometimes; but it will be an empty victory because you will never get your opponent's good will" (Carnegie 122).

Being right, winning an argument, and speaking our truth are distractions. *Impact is about actual change*: i.e., helping the other person become more open to changing his or her mind and acting in a manner that contributes to less animal suffering. If that happens, then it's not just we who win, but everyone.

You may know philosopher Jeremy Bentham's famous dictum, *"The question is not: can they reason? nor: can they talk? but can they suffer?"* To emphasize the importance of impact, here's a homemade variation:

> The question is not:
> "Am I right?", nor "Is this my truth?"
> but **"DOES THIS WORK?"**

Is Meat Murder?

MEAT IS MURDER is a well-known slogan (launched by the band the Smiths two decades ago). It can often be found on buttons and stickers, and as part of vegans' arguments. But is meat *really* murder? Well, not how murder is presently defined. Murder, at this moment, is legally the taking of another human life. It also implies malicious intent, which isn't present in meat eaters or slaughterers (we assume and hope). And do we mean that killing for meat is murder, or that that meat eating itself is murder?

You can see the problems in concluding that "meat is murder" is a true statement. Maybe it's *our* truth and *we* believe it wholeheartedly. But others don't. We may try to convert them, and some people may tell us we're correct. But what we should really care about is not whether meat *is* murder but whether the slogan is effective. Will people be any closer to changing their minds and listening to our arguments, or just annoyed with us when we say it? Do they feel we're accusing them of something and making them feel guilty? Do they think we're holier-than-thou and resent us for making them uneasy and, thus, even less likely to change?

These questions are hard to answer, and we will probably never find out what sort of influence our discussion has on the other person. Indeed, our interlocutor may not even know it him- or herself. Still, it *is* possible to be open to people's response to us, if they are genuinely thinking about what we've said or are defensive; if they like or dislike us, and are enjoying the conversation or not.

Let's make this question, and the dichotomy between speaking our own truth and speaking effectively, more concrete. Imagine someone asks you: *So, do you think I'm a murderer?* I cannot imagine that answering in the affirmative would lead to a fruitful conversation in most cases. ■

It's Not about You, It's about Them

Vegans believe (rightly) that they have an extremely important message and that people should listen. It's my observation that we'll reach them more effectively by *not* making ourselves or our message the center of attention, but the person(s) we're communicating with. If we refuse and say, "No, it's about the animals, not about them!" then we've already fallen into the trap of only being interested in what *we* want—even if it *is* about the animals.

Some people are well trained to focus on others. A therapist will concentrate on her client and vanish into the background. She'll listen attentively, and when she talks it will mostly be to ask questions. As activists, we often behave in the opposite manner. We believe we have a therapy ready that will solve everyone and the world's problems, and people just have to listen to us and apply it.

One of the best books about talking to people, influencing others, and conducting valuable conversations is the timeless classic *How to Win Friends and Influence People* by Dale Carnegie. In spite of its title, Carnegie's bestseller is not about manipulating people, but about being sincerely interested in others. Carnegie puts the need for a focus on our audience like this: "Of course, you are interested in what you want. But no one else is. The rest of us are just like you: We are interested in what *we* want."

Think about who among your friends and family you have the best discussions with. You may like them as conversation partners for different reasons. They may tell interesting stories. They may be hilarious and light up a room. But chances are that the reason you enjoy their company is because they take an active interest in *you*. They ask sincerely how *you* are doing, not as a formality but because they want to know the answer. They want to know what's on *your* mind, and they inquire how they can help *you*. They're people who let you tell *your* story.

We need to be that kind of person if we want others to be open to what we have to say. True, it's perfectly possible to be manipulative. But it's just as possible to be sincerely interested in other people because we care about them, just as we care about animals.

YANYA: YOU ARE NOT YOUR AUDIENCE

A facet of being audience-centered is realizing that we're not necessarily the same kind of people as those we want to reach. "You are not your audience" (I abbreviate it to the principle YANYA) means that whatever applies to you doesn't necessarily apply to your target audience. As a case in point, just because *you* became a vegan after watching the film *Earthlings* doesn't mean that everyone else will, or should. In psychology, the idea that everyone is and thinks like you on a certain issue is called *false-consensus bias.*

People differ from one another in numerous areas, not least in what influences thinking and behavior. We differ in age and education, which may help determine our openness to new ideas or habits. We differ in mental and emotional flexibility, speed of picking up new ideas, and capacity to learn. Some of us are better cooks than others. Some of us have allergies or a chronic condition that may make it more difficult for us to eat a particular diet. Some of us love new foods, others are wary of them. We all experience different childhoods. Most importantly, we're interested in and passionate about different things. Some care about the environment, others about their health, still others about their wallets. Some don't seem to care about anything at all.

One way to see the difference between ourselves and the rest of the population is in terms of the famous "diffusion of innovation" model (see Fig. 13), which tries to explain and predict the rate at which new ideas and technology will spread throughout a population (Rogers).

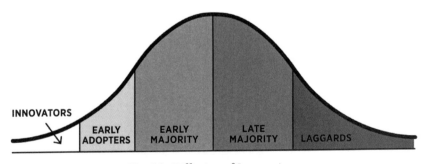

Fig. 13: Diffusion of Innovation

Let's take the smartphone as an example. Look at the innovation curve in Fig. 13 to guess where you're situated. If you live in a technologically advanced country and bought a smartphone in 2005, you were among the innovators or early adopters. If you bought your first smartphone recently (say in 2017), you're in the late-majority category. You're cautious and like to wait until you can be sure. Much as we might like to imagine that all people are innovators (vegans are innovators under this schema), this diagram illustrates that people have different motivations for and concerns about taking on something they consider new. It would be a mistake to try to get the late majority onboard right away with the arguments that influenced the innovators or early adopters.

Remember Solomon Asch's experiment about conformity from the first chapter? The lesson was that many people feel a great need to conform. In their food choices, too, conformists don't want to be perceived as deviating from the norm. Some will wait until it's "safe" to switch to another diet or product. The famous marketer Seth Godin puts it like this: "The mistake idea merchants make is that they bring their fringe ideas to people who don't like fringe ideas, instead of taking their time and working their way through the progression" (2015). Godin suggests changing vocabularies depending on the audience: using words like *new, breakthrough,* or *pioneer* for the innovators; and *proven, established,* or *everyone* to address the rest (2017).

What Godin and others are saying is that we should meet people where they are and appeal to the values they already cherish, rather than telling them which values they *should* have. We're often prone to think that we'll influence people with the arguments that have meant something to *us*. We believe an argument makes so much sense that others would be crazy not to agree with it. But others might not be interested in our arguments or in rational argumentation at all. Especially when it comes to food (and even more so, meat), we can behave deeply irrationally. We'll go out of our way and ignore all kinds of warnings in order to keep eating the food we love and have since childhood, and that we associate with wonderful family moments.

Of course, vegan advocates do have things in common with the audience that we want to reach. Most people care about some animals to some degree. But that orientation is usually not enough motivation to make people change, so that orientation shouldn't lead us too quickly to take the next step and say: *You care about animals so you should not eat meat.* That conclusion is often one bridge too far or a step taken too quickly. The same people who say they love animals may have other values, too—as they may have other concerns, issues, and fears that it would be unwise for us to ignore.

We can try to employ with everyone the arguments that we found convincing. And we blame them if they don't change. But often we'll only

GOTTA HAVE MY JUNK FOOD

On the menu of the Heart Attack Grill in Las Vegas you can find burgers that literally come with a health warning, with names like the "quadruple bypass burger." Waitresses are dressed up as (sexualized) nurses. A morbidly obese man who greeted customers at the entrance died of a heart attack a few years ago. People willingly and knowingly walk into this restaurant to subject themselves to this kind of food.

Another illustration of how irrational people can be around food is what occurred when chef Jamie Oliver introduced a healthy lunch program to some British schools a few years ago. When students at one of those schools continued to eat their usual junk food at the McDonald's or Burger King around the corner, teachers decided not to let the students out during lunch break, so that the healthy (or at least *healthier*) dishes would be their only option. A couple of mothers were so angry at this decision that they took orders from the students through the school fence, went to their favorite fast-food restaurants, and single-handedly brought back about seventy orders for the students each day for the next couple of weeks. These examples make clear that people are irrational when it comes to what they eat. ∎

be kidding ourselves. A better decision would be for us to remember that we are *not* our audience, and to practice what may be the most important skill any activist can develop: to walk in another's shoes.

Walking in another's shoes means that we try to imagine what it's like to be that other person. Who are they and what issues are they dealing with? How do they see our issue and hear our message? What do they focus on? What do they ignore? What sounds incredible, stupid, or unfeasible to them? And, no less importantly, How do they perceive us as the messenger? How credible are we to them? How sympathetic are we, or how annoying?

Walking in another's shoes is a learned skill. Even if we pride ourselves on our empathy, most of us find putting ourselves in someone else's position difficult. Even when we think we're doing it, we can always improve. Some factors may impede our understanding of what it's like to be someone else. We may have class, gender, racial, or other prejudices (and privileges). We may have lived in our vegan bubble for so long we've forgotten what it was like to be an omnivore.

We may find it difficult to understand nonvegans in online discussions because of the limits of the medium, whether those limits are 140 characters, multiple simultaneous threads, or troll-infested feeds. We may get so riled up that we don't even *want* to understand where the other person is coming from. We may say we don't care about how others see, hear, or perceive us. That's a perfect release valve and attitude . . . *if* we have nothing to "sell." Except, of course, we have a *lot* to sell!

Some may think we can only approach others using certain, well-defined techniques, according to a certain ideology or philosophy that outlines clearly what is or is not permissible in our outreach. Some vegans will actually consider it unethical to take into account where other people are and will only want to bring their message in its pure, undiluted form. This is more or less the opposite of walking in other people's shoes. It's the conviction that *other* people should walk in *our* shoes, whether they fit or not and whether they like them or not, because they are the only *correct* pair of shoes.

Car salespeople attempt to get a sense of what potential customers value. They talk about the safety of the car to young parents and emphasize its coolness to single men (pardon the clichés). The salespeople know there's no single "right" argument to sell the car, and they aren't concerned about following the rules and guidelines of the sales textbook they had to study in college. All they know is that they'll be most successful if they

SOME PRACTICE

PLAYING THE DEVIL'S ADVOCATE

An exercise that can help you take another's viewpoint is to play the devil's advocate and try to make a convincing case against your own, either by yourself or in dialogue with someone else. You can argue, for example, that it's a real challenge to go vegan. (Pick anything that you basically disagree with.) If you do this well, you may discover more and/or better arguments than you previously thought existed.

YANYA EXERCISE

Try to imagine what omnivores, and not you as a vegetarian or vegan, might feel about the following statements. Think each one through. You may ask omnivorous friends for their opinion:

- President Bill Clinton being touted as a vegan in the newspaper, but eating fish
- A vegan not wanting to eat a sandwich because it touched a meat sandwich
- Non-Jewish vegans comparing what happens to the animals to the Holocaust
- What people of color think when white vegans compare animal husbandry to slavery
- Vegans refusing to participate in Christmastime or Thanksgiving dinners because dead animals are being served ■

tailor their patter to the audience. Keeping our audience in mind means there isn't one correct approach, but that we should always adapt and see which is the best fit.

THE ART OF LISTENING

What we say may be less important than *how* we say it and the dynamic that emerges between ourselves and the other person. As author Maya Angelou said: "I've learned that people will forget what you said, people will forget what you did, but people will never forget how you made them feel." In the end, the person we're talking to will leave with a certain feeling about the whole interaction. Whether that feeling is positive or not doesn't depend on the arguments we present, but on our whole attitude. Process, in other words, may be more important than content. How friendly were we? Did we let our interlocutors finish? Did we make them feel we understood their arguments or did we talk the whole time ourselves? Maybe the most important question here is: How well did we listen?

Listening skills are profoundly important for advocacy, and for being a pleasant human being in general. Think of those you know who are really bad listeners. They talk all the time, and when you say something it's not clear if they heard you or not. They give no sign that they did. They start on about their own issues immediately. They hardly ever ask questions and, if they do, they don't listen to your answer. Most of us find such people tiring and annoying.

As passionate advocates for the animal cause, we might be even worse at listening than the general population. We have crucial, life-changing information to offer and other people need to shut up and listen to us! We want the world to know all the facts we have at our disposal. We want our audience to understand our arguments and follow and copy our train of thoughts as well as our behavior, preferably without question. Moreover, we believe that whatever our audience will say or object to, we've heard it all before, and there's precious little need to listen to them. Consequently, it's all too simple for us to be self-centered and self-focused, and to lose touch with our audience.

By contrast, people who are good listeners make us feel heard. They recognize us. We feel valued by their attention and their presence. Sometimes, however, when people talk to us about an issue (they may have problems with their significant other or had a fight with their mom or son) we're thinking about what to say, if we're not distracted by other thoughts. But saying something is not always necessary. Our suggestions for solutions may be welcome, but often all that people need is someone who really hears them. In his book *Nonviolent Communication: A Language of Life*, Marshall Rosenberg puts it like this: "Don't just do something, stand there." Rosenberg says that believing we have to "fix" situations and make others feel better prevents us from being present (p. 93). He quotes the psychologist Carl Rogers:

> "When . . . someone really hears you without passing judgment on you, without trying to take responsibility for you, without trying to mold you, it feels damn good! When I have been listened to and when I have been heard, I am able to perceive my world in a new way and to go on. It is astonishing how elements that seem insoluble become soluble when someone listens, how confusions that seem irremediable turn into relatively clear flowing streams when one is heard." (p. 113)

Stephen Covey, author of the bestseller *The Seven Habits of Highly Effective People*, says: "Most people do not listen with the intent to understand; they listen with the intent to reply." It's not necessarily a bad thing to have a ready answer when it's our turn to speak, especially when we're in a public debate, for example. But formulating a response in our head will obviously affect the quality of our listening and thus jeopardize our understanding of the other person.

Listening wouldn't be half as useful if the other person didn't realize you *were* listening. Try this experiment: Tell a conversation partner not to provide you with any verbal or nonverbal cues, such as nodding or saying "uh-uh" or "OK." It's weird and annoying, isn't it? These little feedback expressions are crucial for a conversation. It's also useful now and then to paraphrase what the other person said ("So you're saying that . . . ?"), since that response helps you listen more attentively and makes the other person feel heard. The same goes for asking questions. Of course, none of this should be a mechanical process in which we use paraphrasing and questions to pretend we're listening or empathizing. We have to be genuinely interested in the answers they give.

In *The Animal Activist's Handbook*, Matt Ball and Bruce Friedrich go further and suggest that when people have questions or objections, we consider *answering* these with a question. That may be effective for three reasons: (1) We can make people think; (2) We make them feel heard, and they may return the favor by listening in turn; and (3) From their answers we may learn more information about them (p. 49). The most obvious example of this technique is to answer the question "Why are you vegan?" with "Why do you eat meat?"

Of course, when *we* are communicating, we'd like others to take note. Sharing our opinions, values, and facts with people is far from a waste of time, especially if they ask to hear them. Just remember to pay attention to the process and to listen. And don't overdo it. Consider the *quantity* of information you provide others with. We often think that the more information we give, the better. But it's easy for us to be overwhelming. Besides, people also have a limited ability to listen. They'll get bored or distracted after a while.

How well we listen may involve several factors outside our control. (Namely, some of us may have remarkably short attention spans.) What we should avoid is giving people reasons *not* to listen to us. One technique is not to appear too different from our audience. Meeting people where they are means we have an idea of their desires and objectives and what interests them. It means speaking their language and jargon. It may even mean looking like them. We know from research that how we look influences how credible we are and how people relate to us. This is one further element in which we can be adaptive. If we give a presentation inside a large company, we might choose to dress differently from when we're addressing a crowd at an ecofest. In *Rules for Radicals*, Saul Alinsky gives more drastic advice: "If the real radical finds that having long hair sets up psychological barriers to communication and organization, he cuts his hair." "My thing," Alinsky adds, "is solid communication with people in the community" (p. 19).

The remainder of this chapter consists of more do's to practice and don'ts to avoid in achieving this "solid communication."

TREADING SOFTLY

Understanding others—a prerequisite to enabling them to open their hearts and minds, and thus to helping animals—means comprehending what I call the "big vegan handicap." The term, which I borrow from golf to indicate an initial disadvantage, describes how advocates have to deal with a degree of defensiveness when they talk to people about not eating animals. Activists can attribute the defensiveness to the nonvegan's laziness and indifference. However, I believe it's more productive to examine two other emotions: guilt and fear.

Most vegans have experienced it, often more than once. You're sitting around the dinner table with other people. They know or at some point find out that you're vegetarian or vegan and the conversation turns to not eating meat. Omnivores in this situation often become defensive or angry, even when you're accommodating and open. Vegans need to understand that our mere presence can be enough to make nonvegans uncomfortable. This discomfort will influence the discussion and the nonvegans' attitude.

As I've stated before, I believe that most people are aware that how animals are raised today doesn't accord with the values they consider appropriate for our treatment of them: kindness not cruelty, care and not exploitation. The general public is more or less conscious that pigs, chickens, and cows undergo suffering they'd not wish on their own dog or cat. They may think it would be better to buy "humane meat" (believing there is such a thing), or even that killing animals for food is wrong. Faced with the discrepancy between our beliefs and our actions, many of us feel guilty. Anthropologists have found many examples of premodern civilizations that

TALKING TO A HUNTER

A great example of audience-centered communication is offered by Matt and Phil Letten, the duo known as Vegan Bros. When an individual tells an animal advocate that he or she likes to hunt and asks what we think about it, the Vegan Bros suggest we answer so that the hunter isn't placed on the defensive or assumes we hate her or him. Their suggestion is to say this: "I'm not going to say hunting is good. But it is nowhere near as bad as factory farming." Many animal advocates would consider this a mistake because it appears to condone hunting. Nonetheless, we'd be telling the truth: hunting *is* less bad than factory farming. Framing the conversation in this manner means you shift the conversation to factory farming. When both parties can agree on a topic, you've found a starting point for discussion. Furthermore, the hunter may see us as someone open for discussion and whom they can (on this) relate to. ■

coped with their guilt for killing animals with specific atonement ceremonies (Serpell). Although, unlike these communities, most of us no longer live among the animals we eat, many of us may feel even *more* culpable than we might have done in the past at our thoughtless exploitation.

We vegetarians and vegans are living, breathing reminders of this discrepancy and guilt. We bring up the cognitive dissonance that nonvegans may be trying to quash. "The mere presence of a vegetarian will increase dissonance experienced from consuming animal flesh," writes one researcher based on a study (Rothgerber 37). That nagging interior voice that nonvegans don't want to hear is telling them that they've been behaving unethically, and doing so all their lives.

Realizations such as these aren't fun. As Melanie Joy writes: "Nobody wants to identify with the bad guy, and people will go to great lengths to avoid seeing themselves in a negative light, including refusing to support a cause they might otherwise believe in" (2008, p. 19). In chapter 3 we talked about how people reduce internal conflict (dissonance-reducing strategies) by, in this case, rationalizing meat eating with a variety of arguments, from terrible to weak.

When people see others make more ethical choices they may become resentful and denigrate them—a phenomenon called *do-gooder derogation* (Minson and Monin). In one study, those who shopped for clothes using ethical barometers such as whether the clothes were made in sweatshops were judged by the "willfully ignorant" as odd, less sexy, and unattractive. The thorniest problem here isn't the derogation itself, but that the act of denigrating undermines the denigrator's own commitment to ethical values in the future. The authors claim that the derogation is partially driven by the self-threat that consumers feel when they make a negative social comparison with others (like vegans). Vegans should therefore try to reduce the negative contrasts, which do *not* stimulate people to better-consumption behavior. Instead, the studies' authors suggest, they should "promote a scenario in which consumers are likely to demonstrate moral elevation as opposed to self-protective negative judgments of others" (Zane et al.).

Nonvegans often complain that vegetarians and vegans are preachy and moralizing. Many times that's true, partly perhaps because of the strongly ethical bias within veganism and the philosophical basis of animal advocacy since the mid-1970s. It's also true that vegans, myself included, may talk about "ethical veganism" and refer to "educating others" in a fashion that gives an impression of moral superiority and assumption that those who don't share our views are unschooled.

However, the above study makes clear that nonvegans' complaints about vegan moralizing are driven partly by the nonvegans' defensiveness. To stop nonvegans thinking like this, one thing we vegans can do is to talk about our own imperfections: of the actions we took that we know we shouldn't, or how we didn't become vegan overnight and needed some persuading ourselves. It's vital for vegans to show nonvegans that we're not some kind of alien species with an unattainable level of morality or discipline.

How to Be a Nonjudgmental Vegan

Many of us vegans find it difficult *not* to blame meat eaters, or not to be judgmental—and even harder not to come across as judgmental. Still, we have to try neither to be nor appear so, as most people who feel judged will be less likely to listen and change. In my experience, no one likes a "judger." Here are some tips on avoiding being or seeming judgmental:

- *Grow your self-awareness.* Try to catch yourself when you're being judgmental. Being aware of it is a first step to changing it.
- *Realize that you don't know people or their situation.* Think of something those you're judging might be experiencing. Realizing they may have a good reason for their behavior can calm you in an instant. You may curse a reckless driver in traffic, but what if he's en route to the hospital to visit his dying mother?
- *Remember that everyone is different.* We were reared differently, have a different genetic makeup, lead different lives. Because of these reasons, we do things differently, and may need more time to change.
- *Admit that you're not perfect.* Being a vegan doesn't make you awesome in all aspects of your life. Be wary of throwing stones while living in a glass house.
- *Recall that you (probably) were a meat eater once.* Unless you've been vegan from birth, you may have entertained the same ideas and used the same arguments as nonvegans. (And if you were reared as a vegan, it was not your conscious decision.) Did you go vegan the moment someone told you it was wrong to eat animals? Or were you primed already by your environment?
- *Comprehend that people may be doing great deeds, which you aren't.* They may be helping in a homeless shelter, volunteering

for a human relief organization, or donating money to good causes. You don't have a lock on virtue or compassion.

- *Turn it around. Think of a situation in which someone judges you for stuff you're doing wrong.* How would you react if you met someone who's "more vegan" than you? Or is a vegan *and* a pro-bono human rights lawyer? Try to be honest. You may think you are Ms. or Mr. Rational, who'll admit to being wrong and changing your behavior on a dime. But it's more likely that you'll start to conjure reasons to protect your sense of self-worth.

- *Realize that trying to be nonjudgmental is a matter of effectiveness.* If you can suspend judgment, your activism will be better—for the animals, for the person you're judging, and even for you. ∎

The research on what role guilt plays as a driver for behavioral change is complex. Guilt can definitely lead to change in some circumstances, but we need to be circumspect about mixing it into our vegan messaging. Guilt-based messages can make someone even less likely to do what you want him or her to do, as they're likely to evoke self-protection rather than encourage action (Brennan and Binney).

When I interact with nonvegans, my working assumption is that they already possess a certain (useful) sense of guilt, and that it's not beneficial to strengthen that guilt by talking or writing in an accusatory tone, or suggesting their complicity in horrendous cruelty. I've found it more helpful to provide nonvegans with ideas on how to cope with guilt, which in practice boils down to helping them to avoid eating animals. If we want to blame someone it's better to target the meat industry, without giving the impression that we consumers don't bear any personal responsibility. Melanie Joy talks about "walking the fine line between *challenging* and *supporting* the listener's paradigm" (2008, p. 119).

Next to guilt is fear. Some vegans might find the fears that people express over going vegan ridiculous and trivial compared to animal suffering. I sympathize with that idea, but it's not particularly effective to treat such concerns as simply whining. Put yourself in the other person's shoes and consider what kind of fears they may have—fears you may have long forgotten. There's the fear they'll never enjoy food as much as they do today; of being unhealthy; of no longer being welcome at dinner parties or family celebrations; of mockery and even ostracism from loved ones or humiliation by vegans for being inconsistent when they can't wholly adopt the diet; of losing part of their identity and becoming a different person, among other anxieties.

None of these fears is life-threatening, but none is conducive to change, either. We should try to avoid increasing nonvegans' fears or concerns. It's not constructive, for example, to name every item nonvegans won't be allowed to eat or buy as vegans.

One terrific means of dealing with nonvegans' concerns is the so-called *Feel, Felt, Found* approach, derived from sales. It consists of three steps:

1. Empathize with your listeners. Validate how they **feel**, and really hear their concerns.
2. Reassure your interlocutors by saying they're not the only one to have **felt** like this. Here it is of course important to be in touch with what you felt before you went vegan (or maybe still feel), rather than pretending you never had this feeling. You can also refer to what other people have felt.
3. Let them know what you and others have **found** that is comforting.

Let's say a nonvegan host tells you she loves throwing dinner parties and she's afraid of limiting her cooking by reducing her choice of ingredients. Again, this may sound inconsequential to vegans, but as this *is* a concern to her, you should take it seriously. You could say:

Right, so you feel that going vegan might limit your creativity in the kitchen. I understand that. I felt the same. It's like: What's left, right? And you know, in theory you're certainly right. In practice, most vegans seem to find that once they ditch meat and dairy, they actually increase the variation in their ingredients and cooking. That's because being vegan leads you to discover all kinds of products and ingredients you never knew existed, let alone tasted.

CAN A SUPERLOCAVORE VEGAN MAKE YOU FEEL GUILTY?

It's not easy to walk in other people's shoes and imagine the feelings we may engender in others with our communication. If we don't think guilt is counterproductive, if we don't experience or have forgotten about persuasion-resistance, if we can't imagine being irritated with do-gooders . . . then it's hard to take those feelings into account.

Here's an exercise that can help us be more empathetic regarding those feelings. The point is to imagine someone whose behavior seems even more consistently virtuous than yours—someone who goes beyond veganism. Let me present to you Belle, the superlocavore (SV) vegan (from *locavore*: eating locally). Belle takes into account the fact that in the mechanized harvesting of plants, many small rodents and birds, not to mention insects, are killed. So Belle only eats what she harvests (by hand) from her own organic garden (and those of her fellow SVs). She doesn't purchase anything from stores.

Belle believes her diet is possible for everyone, since those without a garden can find another SV with one and live off that land. She considers her lifestyle the "moral baseline," and that it's an ethical duty to eat as she eats. People who are merely vegan (and hence consume plant products that entailed the avoidable suffering of small rodents and birds) are, in Belle's eyes and those of her friends, hypocrites.

How would you feel if you met Belle and she called you a hypocrite? I'm sure many a vegan would rush to point out to Belle the differences between a vegan and a SV, between cows and those rodents, between intentionally eating animals and eating plants the harvest of which unintentionally killed animals . . . but I'm not sure there truly *is* a difference. If there is, it's small enough for us to suspend our disbelief and go along for a moment with this exercise. The point is to imagine someone like Belle, who can engender a sense of inferiority or guilt within us.

Another example of others being considerably more virtuous are those who donate a percentage of their income to good causes, as the Effective Altruism (EA) movement suggests. William MacAskill, one of the founders of EA, has pledged to give away every penny he earns over £28,000. Think about how much money you earn. Can you see how other people could argue that you need to give some of that away? What if they said it was immoral not to, and that you will be responsible for the deaths of several people if you spend your money on a new cellphone or clothes you don't need rather than on those dying of disease, homelessness, or hunger? ∎

In this response, you've validated your nonvegan host's concern by describing it and by telling her she's not the only one to have it. You've given her a possible answer or solution, not by forcing one on her and telling her how she should feel, but by offering your own positive experience.

In regard to the "big vegan handicap"—the difficult starting position because of nonvegan defensiveness—my suggestion is to go the extra mile to put the omnivore at ease, and not add gasoline to the fire. Whatever we vegans say to our audience may sound more guilt-inducing than we expect or intend. So we need to tread carefully. I don't mean we need to be deferential or overly respectful of people's preferences and sensibilities. Although manners and politeness matter of course, my point is that we will be more successful if we meet nonvegans where they are and appreciate their personal situation. Understanding where they come from may help us develop a much more personalized and thus more effective means of talking to them.

I understand the attractions of not pussyfooting around issues and adopting a wishy-washy attitude. It's satisfying to speak our mind boldly and stand up for what we believe. And with some nonvegans, direct confrontation might work. However, as I argue throughout this book, the main task is to adapt and change our approach according to what we think our audience is attracted. We may not know exactly what that preference is and, with any luck, our audience may be so large that it contains many different sorts of people in it. But my point still holds. In such a scenario, it's best to embrace an approach that we have reason to believe works for the greatest number of people (the lowest common denominator, as it were). In general, when advocates go in blind and have to choose between using a gentle, even sugarcoated message or an in-your-face clarion call, the former is probably the safer and more productive option at this moment in vegan history.

From Why to How, from Theory to Food
When we think of animal advocacy, what comes to mind first are actions like handing out leaflets, talking, or debating. In other words, advocacy to us consists mainly of promoting the reasons *why* (the arguments, moral or not). Talking to people about the *why* often becomes a discussion or a debate. We're trying to use both rational and emotional arguments to change nonvegans' minds, and make them see, understand, and feel what we do. But as many vegans know from personal experience, these kinds of interactions often aren't as productive as we'd like. Not everyone is interested in having a discussion in the first place, and not every situation or place is suitable for a discussion. (Nonvegans may be on the defensive, for example, when they're at a barbecue munching a grilled steak.)

One alternative to a live conversation is to give people a web address, flyer, or book to check out at home. When we read or watch some material privately, we can more easily let our guard down. We don't have to be afraid of losing face and we don't need to try to prove we're smarter than someone else. We're more likely to let the information bypass our resistance and give some time to thinking about it.

Indeed, discussions and debates may not only be unproductive, but may be becoming less and less important. As more and more nonvegans find their information through the Internet and other mass media, they're often quite willing at least to eat or cook vegan meals now and then, but often don't know *how*. When people believe they know *how* to do something, chances are better they'll do it. Psychologists talk about self-efficacy, or a person's belief in his or her capacity to execute behaviors necessary to achieve something (Bandura, Kreausukon et al., Reuter et al.).

Showing nonvegans *how* also contributes to keeping new vegetarians and vegans onboard. Nowhere in all my research did I read that many people stopped being vegetarian or vegan because they no longer believed in the reasons why they became vegetarian or vegan in the first place. Encouraging people on how to keep healthy, cook, locate stores, and find products in them seems therefore essential. Given that one-third of vegetarians lapse after only three months or fewer, this practical information should be handed over to would-be vegetarians from the start. Based on their study of former vegetarians, Faunalytics recommends that we should increase the focus on the *how* of vegetarianism/veganism and "design outreach and supporting efforts to address the most common difficulties" (Asher et al. 2014).

When vegans make veganism more about the *how*, our focus almost automatically shifts to food. Whereas our arsenal of pro-vegan arguments is about theory (the *why*), food is about practice (the *how*). Clearly, food needs to occupy a fundamental place in our outreach. Berthold Brecht once wrote: "Food comes first, then morals." Brecht meant that people worry first about their stomachs, and other material needs, and only subsequently about ethics. Similarly, many nonvegans aren't going to think about animals as long as they feel they'll be missing out on great food. It's easy to imagine the difference between talking to someone who's never had a good vegan taste experience (or worse: someone who's had only had a "bad tofu experience" and is therefore deeply stuck in "veg prejudice"), and someone who knows how great vegan food can be. In the second case, that individual will be much more likely to really listen to pro-animal arguments. As an industry analyst says about vegan companies: "They've got to get this product into people's mouths, then they can talk about all the benefits of it" (Purdy).

By focusing on food, I do not intend to reduce animal rights simply to satisfying taste buds. I'm also not limiting our cause to merely another facet of consumerism or a frivolous search for vegan desserts and cupcakes. I focus on food for three reasons:

1. Food is at the core of animal suffering and killing. By far the greatest numbers of animals we mistreat and kill are for the purpose of food.

2. Food may be our movement's largest asset. Nothing (except perhaps sex) sells like food. It's universally loved, it's easy to attract people with, and it's associated with something positive. So focusing on great food is crucial. This is why VegFund, an organization that provides grants for vegan actions and campaigns, focuses among other things on food-sampling events; or why ProVeg International coordinates the Worldwide Vegan Bakesale in over twenty countries.

3. Food brings people together. It's the social glue for gatherings involving family, friends, coreligionists, or coworkers. Many nonvegans worry about endangering this social dimension and may be wary of vegetarians or vegetarian debates at the table (especially, as noted, during dinners at Christmastime or Thanksgiving), let alone becoming one themselves.

The pivotal role of food for the vegan cause means that cooking for people, eating with them, inviting them out, or helping them have a good vegan food experience isn't just a vital means of communication, it's a great opportunity to provide an alternative to debating and other kinds of oral influencing. If you know you're not a smooth talker or you get too emotional or impatient, you can take to the stove for others. Even if you *are* a wonderful conversationalist, consider cooking as a complementary form of outreach. Have a discussion over a meal you cook or buy for the other person.

With so much vegan information and so many recipes now freely available on the Web, it's tempting for vegans to think that those with no idea of where to start are obtuse or apathetic. However, we should keep in mind that in most Western industrialized countries, we've no tradition of vegan (nor vegetarian) cooking. We've either become rich enough to be able to eat meat at every meal, or we've grown up with processed and not whole foods, or we've lost connections to our ancestral diets where meat was only a condiment.

To that extent, Western societies offer some of the least fertile ground for spreading vegetarian/vegan culture. When I talk to groups of nonvegans, I often ask them to name me one vegetarian (let alone vegan) main course their grandparents or parents put on the table. Except for some poor excuses for main courses (like a hearty soup), most of them come up blank. It's a fair bet that asking the same question in Mexico, India, Japan, China, or Lebanon would present you with many options. It's my conclusion that in richer parts of the world, people who want to go vegan have to relearn how to cook, if they ever learned it in the first place.

On a more structural level, we can develop cooking lessons or help other organizations or institutions to do so, motivate TV channels to start a vegan cooking show, and urge cooking magazines and other publications to include vegan recipes. For those who never cook, or don't have time to cook, we need other tools, which obviously are also useful for the most avid culinary enthusiasts.

A note: Just as in our words and arguments, we can be too idealistic in our food choices. We should offer people the vegan food they want rather than what *we* want to give them. You may be into health foods and believe we all should eat smaller portions, but it's not necessarily the best idea to offer a light salad to someone with a hearty appetite. What's important is that a person likes the food and is satisfied afterward. Don't force your taste in food or cuisine on your new friend; find out what she or he likes and supply it.

Some Ideas to Focus More on the How

My experience of years working for EVA taught me that practical *how* materials (maps of cities, listings of veg-friendly restaurants, recipe booklets, and other communication tools) are much more popular than *why* publications. Here are some tips to make sure we're giving our audience enough *how* information:

- Check your materials and communication for the *how*. Do you devote enough space and time to recipes and nutritional or product information?
- If the answer to the above is *yes*, does it occupy a prominent place on your website and in your materials?
- Does your organization offer cooking courses or provide information on where to find them?
- Temporary vegan pledges or challenges (typically twenty-one or thirty days) are great strategies for sending *how* information to people on a daily basis.
- In one-on-one conversations, experiment with focusing on the *how*. Tell people about the practical steps they can take instead of overloading them with arguments. Invite people not just to read a book or brochure on the problems with animal products, but to shop or cook with you. You can also Friend them on social media. ∎

Toward a More Inclusive Form of Veganism

In this book I've suggested that helping to create a large group of people who reduce their consumption of animal products may be the fastest approach to change the system. Such reducetarian outreach does not replace but complements a go-vegan-for-the-animals strategy. In the following pages, I look at vegans, veganism, and vegan messages. I discuss the *How vegan?* question and the definition of veganism.

Cook It Forward

At EVA we developed a campaign called "Cook It Forward," analogous to the "pay it forward" principle (and movie). With many partners, we offered cooking lessons (including meals) that were free, as long as participants pledged to "cook the meal forward" to at least three other people in their home or somewhere else (who'd do the same). We built a Facebook app to help ensure follow-up. The added advantage to what were essentially cooking lessons was that the concept was so attractive that it was easy to get people enthused about it and to receive commercial sponsoring and government subsidies. ■

The reason I come to this topic so late in the book is because it's contentious. The preceding chapters have offered some arguments and ideas to frame it. One explanation for why it's so contentious is that many vegans are deeply protective of, and identify with, the VEGAN label. This self-identification has positive and negative effects. First of all, I examine the pros and cons of a vegan identity and then suggest a more relaxed concept of veganism as a means of being more inclusive as a movement and thus having a greater impact on behalf of animals.

For many vegans, being vegan is a strong part of our identity. We think about veganism and being vegan a lot. We have vegan friends, visit specialty vegan stores, go to potlucks to meet other vegans, attend vegan talks and conferences, follow vegan Facebook groups, conduct activism together. . . . There's even a word for vegans who want to date only other vegans: *vegansexuals* (Potts).

In a way, creating an identity for oneself is part of what it means to be human. It's entirely natural and perhaps partly necessary to identify with some people, places, objects, and ideas, and to stake a claim that you're a person who loves x, does y, or is against z. An identity and belonging to a group contribute to self-esteem, self-worth, and well-being.

In the case of the vegan movement, creating an identity around veganism has specific advantages. Those for whom veganism is part of their identity may remain vegan longer (Haverstock and Forgays). The Faunalytics research shows that former vegetarians and vegans less frequently consider their diet as part of their identity when compared to current vegans (Asher et al. 2014). In *Vegetarianism: Movement or Moment?*, Donna Maurer writes: "The more a person identifies with a group, the more he or she feels bound by its expectations" (p. 119). In other words, we stick to the rules of our group if we want to keep belonging to it. Undoubtedly, identifying with being a vegan might also make us more committed advocates for our cause: "Sharing a collective sense of who they are helps motivate people to act on their beliefs" (Maurer, p. 119; Van Zomeren et al.). It seems to be easier to derive a sense of identity from a moral ideology than from, for example, concerns for health. Some research (Hoffman et al.) also indicates that ethical vegetarians could experience stronger feelings of conviction and consume fewer animal products than health vegetarians, and remain vegetarian longer.

Veganism as an identity does have important drawbacks, however. An identity can exist only because some people do *not* share it: inclusivity relies on exclusivity. Emile Bruneau, a neuroscientist at M.I.T., has found that people with a strong group identity are less empathic toward an out-group. Talking about sports teams, he says that "the more an individual's team affiliation resonated for [supporters], the less empathy they were likely to express for members of the rival team" (Interlandi).

Now, fans of the Boston Red Sox usually aren't interested in getting fans of the New York Yankees to start rooting for their long-term rivals. In the case of the vegan movement, however, those outside our group are potential allies whom we want to join us. But, as Maurer writes: "If the vegetarian collective identity becomes too strong, vegetarian advocates risk alienating their pool of potential members" (p. 121).

Therefore, two contradictory forces or ambitions are at work in the vegan or similar movements. On the one hand is the ambition to be inclusive. We want to reach out to as many people as possible and persuade them to join us in Veganville. On the other, we wish to build an identity for ourselves, which supplies our group with advantages in retaining members and advocacy.

One solution to this problem for vegans may lie in our distinguishing two different audiences and tailoring our message to them. Vegans should approach the great mass of nonvegans with practical information rather than with the demand that they espouse a vegan identity. We can hardly expect nonvegans immediately to accept all our beliefs and principles. Seeing these as fundamental to "going vegan" only enlarges the magnitude of the call to action and makes entrance to our club unnecessarily difficult and costly. Inviting people to eat vegan food and meals and try vegan products is much easier, for both parties, than asking them to become a vegan or adhere to veganism.

As for the second audience: The vegan identity could be developed among those already vegetarian or vegan, who, if they identify with the movement more, may be motivated to act. Two caveats: Identity can be formed around belonging to a club, but that doesn't mean the club admission price should be astronomically high. Secondly, vegans should be mindful not to derogate or alienate the out-group.

Unfortunately, not only is it common for vegans to alienate nonvegans, but we often alienate our own in-group—or at least, those who to outsiders appear to belong to our in-group. I've long been surprised at how otherwise similar individuals and groups of people take offense at relatively small differences between them. Differences between vegans and vegetarians, or between those who are vegan for ethical reasons and those who stopped eating animal products because of concerns for their health, not only *look* small to outsiders, but *are* small in the grand scheme of things. Still, tension can rise at times between these groups. Freud talks about the "narcissism of small differences." He may not have been describing vegans, but the phenomenon can be discerned everywhere. This is how a psychology textbook explains what is happening:

> People like to be seen in terms of identities important to them. Being seen in terms of other identities, especially erroneous ones, can evoke

"categorization threat." We also do not like it when another group is so similar to ours, because it undermines the very essence of what our group is that makes us different and special. In other words we tend to be most sensitive when the other group actually is similar to our own. . . . Groups that are too similar to our own can therefore threaten the unique identity of the group: "distinctiveness threat." Some have even argued that having a distinctive group identity is even more fundamental than avoiding a negative one. (Hewstone et al.)

If we vegans think it's essential to protect our distinct identity, it's not unthinkable that on a less conscious level some of us may be disturbed if membership in our vegan club gets *too* numerous. Maybe we worry the VEGAN label might lose some of its value when "too many" people acquire it. Perhaps we won't feel special enough any longer and our sense of self-worth will be lowered. It's conceivable that we don't want entrance to our in-group to become so cheap that anyone can join. To an outside observer it might even appear that we don't want to make it easier to help animals, especially if newcomers or new ideas won't have to struggle heroically against the norm as we did.

All such thoughts may not be intentional, but we should be self-aware enough to ensure that we're not raising the price of membership for the sake of safeguarding our identity and self-worth. We should want everyone to join the vegan club. We should want to be as inclusive as possible.

RULES AND RESULTS

If vegans want to be inclusive and welcome everyone to the vegan club, we should be mindful of how we define the rules for admittance. We don't want to make group membership meaningless, but we also don't want it to be too hard. So who ideally can join the vegan club?

To tamper with the definition of veganism is to court controversy. Many vegans will state that veganism already has a clear definition and that there's no reason to tinker with the concept. The terms *vegan* and *veganism* were coined by Donald and Dorothy Watson, cofounders of the Vegan Society in the UK. To rely on an ancient definition as an eternal

> ### Why Fashionable Veganism Is a Good Thing
>
> Some vegans are worried when they see vegan (they would prefer saying "plant-based") diets become more and more associated with health, fun, fashion, or even consumerism, at the cost of their association with ethics. They worry that veganism is devolving into something that's only about diet, eating cupcakes, and exchanging recipes. Veganism, the argument goes, is not a diet, it's a morally infused lifestyle.
>
> I believe a kind of "lighter" veganism is something to champion. We need to reach a situation where being a vegan is so easy that everyone can do it, even those who aren't die-hard animal rights activists, or "health nuts" for that matter. So why complain when some people don't breathe animal rights with every step they take? Since attitude can follow behavior, there's a great chance that these people will "get" the animal rights arguments later. We should allow people to discover the morally good life—something each of us is on an eternal quest to find, moral baselines or not—in steps. ∎

truth isn't necessarily best practice. But even if you're one of those who believe that a founder's definition is, by default, decisive because he or she coined the word, you should realize just how pragmatic the Watsons' veganism was.

The Watsons defined veganism as "a way of living which seeks to exclude, as far possible and practical, all exploitation of animals." On the face of it, this vague and subjective phrasing provides some flexibility. Often, however, I see vegans defining what they deem "possible and practical" not only for themselves, but for everyone else—thus erasing the leeway that the Watsons built into the definition and practice. In essence, many vegans expect of themselves and others complete abstention from animal products. Being vegan becomes like pregnancy: being 97 percent vegan is as impossible as being 97 percent pregnant. Under such logic, if you don't wholly avoid nonvegan foods and products, you cannot call yourself a vegan. For such vegans, clarity and consistency override any attempts to admit that veganism can sometimes be contextual and neither possible nor practical, and such arguments are met with firm opposition. This absolutism is unfortunate, because defining veganism as the total avoidance of animal products—always and everywhere—sets the bar unnecessarily high for nonvegans.

Now, consistency *can* be valuable. Parents will do their best to be consistent in rearing their children, so the latter will know what behavior is acceptable or unacceptable. Philosophers try to come up with theories that are internally consistent, rather than arbitrary or indefensible. For some, consistency and adhering to rules provide discipline and help them avoid what's sometimes called "decision fatigue," or, more seriously, self-destructive behaviors. However, making consistency the sine qua non of our behavior and consumption is misguided. As Ralph Waldo Emerson puts it: "A foolish consistency is the hobgoblin of little minds."

Avoiding the consumption of animal products is a means to an end, which is the minimizing of animal suffering, killing, and injustice. When we're no longer thinking critically about rules and they become the goal, they ossify into dogma. Dogma is dangerous as it forbids critical thinking and resists adaptation to changing times, better ideas, and new information. I'm sure you know someone whom you consider dogmatic. It's not an attractive quality, and has little recruiting power. If we don't want to be dogmatic, we shouldn't blindly follow rules to the letter in all circumstances, but should examine the consequences of our actions.

An example from religious practice may help to show the difference between rules and goals more clearly. When vegans avoid eating animal products, they do so—in part—because they believe this boycott helps animals. When many observant Muslims or Jews, on the other hand, avoid consuming pig meat, most do so because it's a religious mandate. They follow a rule that defines who they are: a Muslim or Jew doesn't eat pigs. Now it may be that rules such as these had their origins in rational considerations. Raising pigs, it turns out, is resource intensive, and so among nomadic peoples in the deserts of the Middle East pigs may have competed with humans for food, and this fact ended up as a religious injunction against raising and eating them. However, Jews or Muslims avoid pig meat today not because of the past goal of leaving enough for humans to eat, but because it's a rule within their religion to do so.

Following rules or sticking to principles in itself is not necessarily harmful . . . until it is. When following rules has no consequences, it can be a waste of energy. When following rules has negative consequences, it may be stifling, distracting, and unproductive.

If we believe following the rules and sticking to our principles (an idealist position) is most important, then we'll support complete consistency as vegans, and may forbid the less observant from using the word *vegan*. If, on the other hand, we look more at consequences (a more pragmatic position), consistency is only of relative importance. After the call for action, the arguments we use, and the environment we help create, consistency is the fourth domain in which we can be pragmatic.

WHY CONSISTENCY IS OVERRATED

My suggestion to enlarge membership of the vegan club is to make the concept of veganism more elastic. If that means that people who aren't completely consistent call themselves vegan, then so be it. The line between vegan and not-vegan may blur, but surely we can tolerate a certain fuzziness if it allows more people to move toward our position. We'll also stop spending so much time and energy policing the borders.

Consider this: Isn't it acceptable for someone to call herself a vegan who doesn't eat animal products except for a slice of her grandmother's pies three times a year? Now, we can certainly question why the man who eats eggs every other day would want to call himself a vegan, but other things we can debate. Here, too, religion is instructive, since all religions contain devotees who are more or less observant and have different beliefs and behaviors, but possess certain core practices and beliefs that they all share. Like vegans, they may also fight over definitions, which is itself instructive of the attractions and distractions of dogma.

Rather than downplaying the importance of being vegan, I want to create some relative perspective and compare the effect of our own vegan consumption with the importance of our communication. Thanks to observing your disciplined and thoughtful vegan lifestyle, you will spare a number of animals a life of suffering. However, the impact you can generate by influencing other people to change their behavior is potentially many times greater.

Consider your friend Jackie. Her veganism isn't as consistent as yours, but she's a real communicator. She blogs, cooks for others, and even starts a business selling animal-free products. It's a good bet that Jackie's "almost-veganism" has potentially a much greater effect than either of your individual practices combined. The illustration below (Fig. 14) represents the relative consequences of what we eat compared to the difference we can make on what others eat.

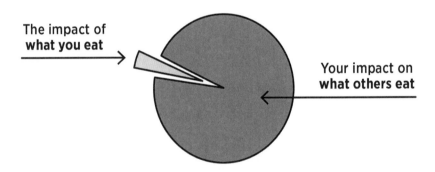

Fig. 14: Your Impact on Animal Suffering

Another significant aspect that can increase our effectiveness is money. Our donations can go far in saving lives, and potentially make a much bigger difference than our own consumption. The website Animal Charity Evaluators (animalcharityevaluators.org) estimates that a $100 donation to one of its most highly recommended charities, The Humane League, will spare the lives of anywhere between 310 and 6,100 animals. The exact number, in view of such a range, is open to debate, but the principle is important: a donation of $100 to help cover the costs of printing flyers may quite possibly save more animals than your many years of not consuming meat and dairy. Incidentally, as donating is so important, we should try to create more of a culture of giving within our movement. Those who do give should advertise their donations, to show others that it's normal and that many of us are doing it. (I'm providing 10 percent of my income to causes that seek to end animal abuse and global poverty.)

Now that we've got some perspective, let me present why I believe that following rules to the letter and being entirely consistent as a vegan is ineffective, unnecessary, insufficient, and impossible—and why allowing for some flexibility may, in fact, work miracles. I want to stress that my aim is to help my fellow vegans compare the model of our own vegan consumption with the importance of how we communicate that vegan model.

BEING WHOLLY CONSISTENT IS INEFFECTIVE

If how we communicate our veganism is potentially so much more powerful than our own consumption habits, we should consider the effect that a perception of strictness may have on those who aren't yet vegan.

In my case, I rigorously inspect the ingredients of whatever I buy in the store. When I'm in public, however, I may occasionally make small exceptions or set aside my doubts about a product or a dish. I don't want to give the impression that being a vegan is more socially prohibitive than it is. Although I'd never knowingly buy or order such products, I can imagine, for instance, eating a veggie burger that might be bound with a small amount of egg, or that may contain a smidgeon of mayo, whey, or casein. Nor will I inquire about the ingredients of wine or bread (knowing the waiter is unlikely to have the answer to my question anyway).

Here is a more concrete example: suppose a nonvegan acquaintance (let's call her Yvonne) took the time and effort to cook me a vegan lasagna as her first vegan cooking experiment, and I found out that Yvonne had inadvertently used pasta made with eggs. No matter how skillfully or diplomatically I might communicate my principles, it's more than likely that Yvonne would end up with a negative perception of veganism. Unlike some vegans, I don't believe Yvonne will so admire my principled stance that she'll be motivated to go vegan. (Remember do-gooder derogation?)

In my judgment, therefore, my *not* eating Yvonne's pasta is more damaging to the animals' cause than eating it. In participating in the meal, I remain true to the goal underlying veganism itself, which for me is the avoidance of suffering and killing. One could, of course, take such accommodations to an absurd limit, and that is not my intention. In my case, simple physical disgust at a slice of cheese would make it impossible for me to make larger exceptions to my principles.

Another example: I know of several people in leadership positions in animal groups who frequently have work lunches with politicians in order to lobby them. These lunches take place in parliament, where no vegan options are available. In order to avoid appearing overly doctrinaire in the politician's eyes, these activists momentarily lower their standards and will eat a vegetarian meal, for pragmatic reasons.

Whereas complete consistency for a vegan can be difficult in private and uncomfortable in public, asking others to be so can be even more problematic. To my knowledge, no research has been conducted on how omnivores perceive principled vegans, nor have studies been undertaken on whether omnivores would embrace veganism if they didn't have to commit to it absolutely and forever. If you're like me, you've heard many nonvegans tell you they could imagine themselves not eating animal products. . . except for that *one* dish they just love *sooooo* much. What if the vegan response to such people was to permit them to make exceptions? Wouldn't the concept of veganism be more accessible? As our metaphor goes: What if we would allow people to leave Veganville now and then?

Jack Norris, director of Vegan Outreach, says: "If people tell me they could go vegan except for the cheese, I tell them to go vegan except for the cheese!" Many of us believe that were we to follow Norris' example, we'd be implicitly condoning something that's unethical. This may be our truth, and it may be consistent with our ideology, but is it effective? As

Henry Spira says: "If you ask for all or nothing, you usually end up with nothing." The point to make here is that our "cheese vegan" (let's call her Emily) would reduce over 95 percent of her "animal suffering footprint." Moreover, I believe Emily's dietary position would at some point lead her to conclude that she doesn't need cheese anyway or it doesn't feel right anymore—not least because she's trying so many phenomenal vegan cheeses that she forgets the "real" kind forever.

Do we vegans really mind if people who eat cheese once a month while the rest of their consumption is vegan call themselves vegan? Would we be wrong to quibble if they called themselves "95 percent vegan"?

My point is that it's more encouraging for people working toward veganism to be included in "our" group, than for us to exclude them a priori because they're not fully vegan yet. The latter position may prevent the would-be vegans from doing anything at all. In other words, vegans should prefer people who act positively inconsistently rather than act negatively with righteous consistency. Calling vegetarians hypocritical or inconsistent may motivate *some* to take the next step, but many others will feel discouraged and alienated. Jonathan Safran Foer puts it well: "We have to get away from the expectation of perfection because it really intimidates people who would otherwise make an effort. People use the fear of hypocrisy to justify total inaction" (Levitt).

Hal Herzog offers a similar example. He quotes a woman who used to be vegetarian. As she didn't seem to be thriving, she went to her doctor, who recommended she eat some form of meat. This doctor obviously was not well informed. Nonetheless, instead of making the minimal concession that her doctor suggested, the patient thought it would be hypocritical to eat one kind of animal and not another. She says: "I went from no meat to all meat" (p. 200). In this case not only was the perfect, as Voltaire writes, the enemy of the good, but the woman's absolutist tendencies pushed her in completely the opposite direction.

We often meet people who tell us they're vegan and then demonstrate some commitment to an animal product. Our response is, usually, to call that person out, but this seems counterproductive to me. I'm sure there are some self-proclaimed vegans who'll thank you for pointing out their inconsistency, but it's my bet that a vast majority would feel alienated and angry.

Let's consider the results if vegans didn't allow almost-vegans to call themselves vegan. We'd be an even smaller club. Those who are vegan 98 percent of the time are, for all practical purposes, vegan, or they're much closer to being a vegan than vegetarian. Letting them signal their vegan identity to researchers, politicians, the industry, or their friends and family seems much more important than avoiding the definitional "confusion" that some vegans seem to fear so much.

A further advantage to being more relaxed about the concept of veganism is that it may help people remain vegan (or almost-vegan) longer. We've already talked about how some people need strict rules about their diet in order to maintain it, whereas others give up because they find sustaining that lifestyle too hard. Of the former vegetarians and vegans in the Faunalytics study, 43 percent indicated they felt it was too difficult to be "pure" with their vegetarian or vegan diet (Asher et al. 2014). That word *pure* ought to tell vegans that the higher our expectations of ourselves and others, and the more vegan rules we invent, the harder it will be to be a vegan.

In an appearance on the Tim Ferriss podcast, journalist Ezra Klein talked about how, whenever he'd fail at being vegetarian, he'd completely collapse into full-on omnivorism. "The reason," Klein says, "in part was that if I'd set up the success structure such that I was vegetarian or I was not, then 'was not' was almost the same kind of failure, no matter how much meat I was eating." Klein tells us about a more successful approach (and identity!) he developed (here about being vegetarian, but it applies also to being vegan):

> The way I went vegetarian a couple of years ago now, was with a tremendous number of caveats: I'm vegetarian except when I travel, because I know when I travel I often have a lot of trouble sticking to vegetarianism; so, if I'm vegetarian except when I travel and then when I travel I eat meat, well then, it doesn't offend my identity at all. And now, I'm mostly vegan. I eat vegan at home, except when I travel I'm vegetarian.

Hypocrites!

When we spot inconsistency in others, we sometimes accuse them of being hypocrites. Vegans may call vegetarians hypocrites because they drink milk, vegetarians may call omnivores hypocrites because they love their dog but eat pigs, and omnivores may call vegetarians and vegans hypocrites for every discrepancy they notice.

I suggest deleting the word *hypocrite* largely from our vocabulary. First of all, the word in these cases isn't correctly used. Hypocrites are those who don't walk their talk, who practice differently from what they preach. If I say to someone he shouldn't hit his children although I hit my children myself, then I'm a hypocrite. If I'm not eating animal products but wearing leather shoes, I may at most be accused of inconsistency. (Wearing leather shoes and telling other people not to wear them would be hypocritical.)

Secondly, the word has a serious, negative moral judgment. We'll endear ourselves to no one by using that word. Venting may make us feel good, but it's usually fruitless. ∎

And, there are a couple of points in the year, like I've been having sushi with my best friend's mother since I was a kid, and it is important to me that I am able to continue that tradition. And so, as opposed to having sushi there twice a year and then collapsing out of all my other eating habits because of it, this is now built into it. And so, I actually find that personally very helpful to not be so strict on myself. (Ferris)

We need more people like Ezra Klein in our movement, not least because Klein is a super-communicator. The more vegans, vegetarians, and reducers there are, so demand for and production of animal products will decrease and fewer animals be raised and killed for food. Some of our choices as vegans make a positive difference, and some are without consequence. But others are harmful. I'd like to think it's obvious where our efforts should lie.

BEING WHOLLY CONSISTENT IS UNNECESSARY

Being strict sometimes has no tangible consequences. The idea behind veganism is a boycott, and the idea of a boycott is to alter demand, which we will have if there are enough of us participating. When an action has no effect on demand, we may still consider the action we're protesting to be morally wrong, but should realize that our boycott is insignificant in the real world. For instance, when you eat something that would otherwise be thrown away or go to waste. In our kitchen pantry sits a box of pasta with eggs that someone accidentally brought. It's has been sitting for quite some time, and my girlfriend and I are wary of eating it, but one could well wonder why, as our eating it will have no impact on demand whatsoever.

BEING WHOLLY CONSISTENT IS INSUFFICIENT

Being a hundred percent vegan is not free of exploitation or cruelty, either for human or nonhuman animals. Not all vegan products are produced locally by well-paid workers. Some are picked by migrant labor or flown from the other side of the world, and climate change causes a lot of human and animal suffering. Some vegan products may still lead to animals suffering directly—from harvesting, monocultures, chemicals, herbicides, and other injuries. Obviously, this knowledge should encourage vegans to be more aware of our food choices rather than to throw up our hands and return to thoughtless omnivorism. Yet a little humility wouldn't go amiss. Veganism, like everything else in this world, is imperfect.

BEING WHOLLY CONSISTENT IS IMPOSSIBLE

The idea that we can be entirely consistent at anything is delusional. In our case, the use of animals for human purposes is so pervasive that it's currently impossible to avoid it absolutely. Consider the spectrum of animal ingredients in Fig. 15 on the next page.

This is an arbitrary collection of nonvegan products or ingredients, ranked according to what probably most vegans can agree is an order of importance. To the left end of the spectrum, we can add hundreds

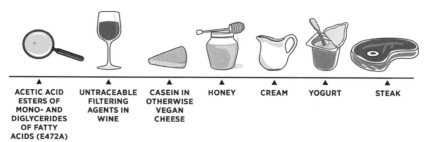

▲	▲	▲	▲	▲	▲	▲
ACETIC ACID ESTERS OF MONO- AND DIGLYCERIDES OF FATTY ACIDS (E472A)	UNTRACEABLE FILTERING AGENTS IN WINE	CASEIN IN OTHERWISE VEGAN CHEESE	HONEY	CREAM	YOGURT	STEAK

Fig. 15: Animal Products on a Spectrum

PRINCIPLES VERSUS CONSEQUENCES:
SOME MORE THOUGHT EXPERIMENTS

I once stumbled across a website (now vanished) that encouraged omnivores to double their meat intake to compensate for the vegans (I kid you not). Far-fetched though this idea was and is, let's entertain the notion that if you go vegan, someone else will commit to eating twice as many animal products. Your consumption behavior in itself would produce no tangible net benefits, since as many animals would suffer and be killed. If, hypothetically, you knew this was happening, would you still remain vegan?

You might remain vegan because, like me, it feels like the right thing to do, or because you're disgusted with meat. However, let's extend the hypothesis to imagine that every time a person turns vegan, an omnivore commits to eating *three* times as many animals. Now the effect of our veganism isn't neutral: it's actually negative. In such a case even I might be tempted to return to eating animal products, as my veganism would bring more suffering into the world.

A related thought experiment that asks you to value principles or consequences is the following: Would you eat a steak for $100,000? You could give that money to an animal rights or pro-vegan organization and they could use it to save a lot of animals. Let's say that no one would see you consume the steak. Or that the steak was going to be thrown away and eating it would have no impact on demand. Would you then?

Finally, here's a more realistic situation. In order to film videos on factory farms and in slaughterhouses, activists go undercover and may need to break some of their own rules so as not to blow their cover. They may need to eat or taste meat or helplessly stand by and watch as animals are mistreated or killed. Does anyone really think these people are bad vegans? They make that compromise because they expect their footage to be influential in helping animals.

These issues, as you may have gathered, are about the question of the ends and the means. To quote Saul Alinsky: "That perennial question, 'does the end justify the means?' is meaningless as it stands; the real and only question regarding the ethics of means and ends is, and always has been, 'Does this *particular* end justify this *particular* means?'" (p. 24) ■

of other ingredients made from animal products that are found in food, cosmetics, and many other kinds of household products.

Now everyone (whether self-defined vegan or omnivore) finds him- or herself somewhere on this spectrum. You may avoid the steak, yogurt, and cream, but be less punctilious about honey, casein, and food additives. You may eat the steak, but draw the line at tucking into frog, dog, dolphin, whale, sparrow, or elephant. The pertinent question is: At what point does one become a vegan, and at what point does one cease to be one? The question becomes yet more complex if we take into account the *quantity* of the substance as well as the *frequency* with which it is consumed. Does Kevin have his vegan badge ripped from his lapel if he consumes a trace of casein once a year? What if Kevin regularly eats nondairy cheese with casein?

We all draw a line somewhere, and for every vegan you'll find someone more hardcore, like Belle, our superlocavore. *Veganissimo A to Z: A Comprehensive Guide to Identifying and Avoiding Ingredients of Animal*

Origin in Everyday Products, by Lars Thomson and Reuben Proctor, consists of over *three hundred pages* of ingredients that are or may be of animal origin, the first element of which is the acetic acid of our example. (It's used in food and can have either mineral or animal sources.) Does being a vegan mean knowing them all by heart and examining each product for any or all of them? What are we to do about ingredients that may not be listed, or could come from animal, mineral, vegetal, or microbial sources?

In her TED talk "How Pig Parts Make the World Turn," Christien Meindertsma explains the incredible range of uses that pig ingredients are put to. They are not just in food products and cosmetics (even before you've had breakfast, Meindertsma says, you've already met the pig many times), but they may also be in buildings, train brakes, china, sandpaper, cigarettes, and more.

It becomes still more complicated when veganism broaches on subjects such as riding a horse or looking after companion animals and buying food for them. Or eating eggs from rescued hens whom you care for in your back yard, or whether you continue to wear your ten-year-old leather shoes. And I've not even touched on whether veganism necessitates the adoption of certain political ideologies, or judgments about abortion, or various ascetic practices. Many vegans will recognize their compromises in these conundrums. What we should ask ourselves, however, is whether we need to make these compromises so definitionally problematic and therefore veganism more difficult.

I do not want to create a "gotcha" or strawman argument. I do realize that even the most vegan of vegans will not suggest that we spend a lifetime studying and avoiding animal ingredients. What I want to illustrate is that some fuzziness is inherent in the concept of veganism, and that there is no clear black and white.

COUNTERARGUMENTS

In the interests of fairness, I can sympathize with those vegans for whom deviating from the trusted concept of veganism as *no* animal products *ever* may feel immoral or offensive. We've already described many of these in the book, but it's worth briefly rehearsing them again, since they're so pervasive and should be addressed directly.

IF WE'RE NOT CONSISTENT, PEOPLE WILL BE CONFUSED

One fear some vegans share is that, without clarity or consistency, vegans are in danger of confusing the public into thinking that veganism is an arbitrary lifestyle instead of a moral imperative.

I feel this argument misses the forest for the trees. In most countries, vegans constitute barely one percent of the population. It's a luxury for vegans to worry about moral imperatives when the vast majority of people haven't even taken the first step toward veganism. It's not important that people are completely clear about what veganism entails; what is, is that they should *move*. As Matt Ball says: "I've never met anyone who, honestly, continued to eat animals because they were confused by a vegan's supposed lack of 'consistency.' What I have seen (and sadly been the cause of) are vegans whose self-righteousness and obsessiveness gave others an excuse to ignore the animals' plight" (Ball, p. 96).

Some vegans worry that a lack of clarity about veganism will mean that waiters and chefs may serve us an animal product (or even lie about a dish) and family members may start to assume we're as casual about our veganism. I'd rebut these concerns, first, by saying that if I'm correct about the greater consequence a more relaxed concept of veganism will have, then dealing with such situations is a small price to pay. We can still communicate what we do or don't want, and should something "wrong" slip into our food, I hope we'd be mature enough to remember that veganism is not about our own purity but about creating real change for animals. Secondly, I'd reiterate that *vegan* as a term is much more usefully and productively applied to dishes and products than people. It's easy to make a dish or product that's wholly vegan. It's much harder to *be* one hundred percent vegan.

WE RISK WATERING DOWN THE CONCEPT OF VEGANISM

Some vegans fear that reducetarian and near-vegan messages will bring us a reducetarian and near-vegan world, where some animals are still exploited. But the nightmare of slippery slopes and a watered-down veganism is a fever dream, and shouldn't concern vegans at the moment. Do we honestly think that a 97-percent vegan world wouldn't be an astonishing improvement over what we live in now? Obviously, we want not a single animal to suffer and be killed for our needs. But by the time vegan meals are the exception rather than the rule, not only will awareness of animal issues be considerable (since we're no longer dependent on using and eating them) but there will be tremendous pressure to eliminate those final percentages.

Micro-ingredients as well as fish, dairy, and eggs will likewise be uneconomical, inefficient, synthesized, or human-made out of existence. We shouldn't worry about the last percentages. The details will take care of themselves. We should get people to take the first, substantial steps. In the meantime, concerned vegans can find support in the fact that more and more vegan organizations are managing to sell their own vegan-certification scheme to companies, thus helping to make sure products that are touted as vegan are really entirely free of animal ingredients.

WE NEED TO SET AN EXAMPLE FOR PEOPLE

Does complete consistency set an example that people want to follow, or could vegans' obsession with it create too great of a distance between vegans and nonvegans? What if it were not only true that you don't need to be vegan to help animals, but, in some situations, nonvegans might actually be better positioned than vegans to inspire other people?

My home country of Belgium hosts a hugely successful campaign on a shoestring budget called Days without Meat. The idea is to avoid meat in the forty days before Easter. The campaign isn't about religion but tags on to Lent as a period in which people try something different, as an experiment or a challenge. In 2017, 115,000 participated in the campaign, which is no small feat for a population of only six million. The initiator is Alexia Leysen, a young woman who is "not even" a vegetarian, but who's reduced her meat intake because of concern for the environment. Now, some vegans might fault her for not being vegan, but the campaign's strength lies in precisely the fact that an omnivore is addressing other omnivores. Everyone is "in it together." There's no vegan from on high telling them what to do or to be like.

In the US, Brian Kateman has initiated the reducetarian campaign, urging people to become a reducetarian and eat less meat (reducetarian. com). In this case, too, it might be good that Kateman is a reducetarian himself. He's not only in a more "equal" position and able to avoid part of his audience assuming he has a holier-than-thou attitude, but his diet permits him to be similar to his audience, which seems to be a factor that helps determine your influence over them (Berscheid, Eagly). (See "The Art of Listening" on p. 125.)

As a final example, British actor and comedian Ricky Gervais comes to mind. Gervais regularly speaks up for cats and dogs, and animals who are hunted or killed for fur. Since he's advocating for more popular animal

PR DISASTER

Just how misguided some vegans are about omnivores' perceptions of (in)consistency became clear to me when the Vegan Society elected a new ambassador a few years ago. Apparently, she wasn't as vegan as some vegans wanted her to be. A Facebook poster defended criticism of her by arguing that the vegan movement had enemies and was under intense scrutiny. The poster reasoned that if these enemies discovered that a Vegan Society ambassador wasn't really vegan, it could turn into a "PR disaster." In my view, the only people who could ever make this into a PR disaster were the vegans who wanted to attack the Vegan Society for their choice of ambassador. Talk about missing the forest for the trees! ∎

causes than veganism, Gervais' large following may be more inclined to listen to him. Imagine that a few years later, he or another such celebrity becomes a vegan and starts addressing farmed-animal issues. Any positive receptivity to the vegan message from the celebrity's fan base will probably be partly due to that celebrity's previous nonvegan stance. If celebrities were as strict as some of us vegans would like them to be, it's likely that many fewer people would listen to them when they spoke on the topic of eating animals.

CONCLUSION: HOW TO BE VEGAN WITH MAXIMAL IMPACT

The vegan movement needs to be inclusive rather than exclusive. We need to think less in terms of us versus them, and more in terms of simply *us*. We share common aspirations and goals with many nonvegans, and if we choose to focus on those instead of our differences and communicate what we'd like in a more generous and welcoming manner, we can grow much faster.

What isn't well known about the Watsons and their fellows at the Vegan Society is that they welcomed everyone who agreed with organization objectives, whether they practiced veganism or not: "An Associate [of the Vegan Society] makes no promise as to behaviour but declares himself in agreement with the object. The door is thus widely opened, and the Society welcomes all who feel able to support it" (IVU). What's interesting here is the distinction between the actual practice of veganism (i.e. not consuming animal products) and accommodating the idea.

Our movement could advance so much further and faster if we considered a part of our team not just those traditionally defined as vegans, but everyone who agrees on the direction—even though they, for whatever reason, may not yet be entirely putting their thoughts and beliefs into practice. This is also why the organization ProVeg International is named as it is: being pro-vegan is emphasizing the direction, rather than the position. It's about being open to all kinds of allies. Being vegan is about helping animals and making sure there is less suffering and killing in the world. There is no all or nothing to that.

If we want a concept of a "real vegan," then I suggest it shouldn't be based on complete avoidance of animal products, but also on the influence we have on others.

If we want a definition of veganism, I suggest we take the Watsons' as the basis, but amend it to be about avoiding animal products insofar as practical, possible, *and effective.*

If we want to be consistent, I suggest we aim to be consistent in the first place not with the rules, ideology, and definition, but with the compassion and ambition to reduce suffering, killing, and injustice, which are the values underlying veganism.

If we need to separate allies from enemies, I suggest we consider as allies those who are looking in the same direction as we are, and who largely agree with the objective, even though they aren't yet entirely walking the talk. And we should also seek the assistance of those not even agreeing with our objectives, but have other motivations for working on solutions that are helpful for us.

After all, we can't do this alone. 🌍

6

SUSTAINABILITY

How to Keep on Keeping On

"Progressive activists are the world's most precious resource."
—**Hillary Rettig**

When a person finally decides to live permanently or semi-permanently in Veganville, our work with them is still not done. At any time, and for different reasons, our travelers may decide to turn back and live somewhere lower on the mountain, or even return whence they came. Just as realistically, we—the same people who've been laboring to get people into Veganville—may at some point become tired of our efforts and burn out.

At some point, we'll be safe. When almost everyone lives in Veganville, it's a fair bet that virtually no one else will consider leaving to live on the otherwise desolate plains below. But until then, we have our work cut out for us.

This chapter is about the sustainability of both being a vegan *and* a vegan advocate. Vegans can return to omnivorism; activists may burn out, and do the same. Below are some ideas about what can be done to prevent this from happening.

KEEPING VEGANS VEGAN

As we've seen, a large number of vegetarians and vegans—no less than 84 percent—at some point stop being vegetarian or vegan (Asher et al. 2014). In chapter 3, I argued that this statistic is less terrifying than it might sound. Still, it would obviously be preferable for there to be more vegans, and for those who are vegans to remain so. As they say in sales, it's a lot easier to keep a current customer than to find a new one.

To tackle this problem, vegans need to take people seriously. It won't help us to blame those who think veganism is too difficult to maintain for selfishness or a weak will. Nor will it help animals if we repeat ad nauseam just how easy veganism is. Instead, we'd do well to really *listen* to nonvegans and be open to their concerns, questions, and observations. Not only will they feel heard, but we may actually be able to help them. The main reasons why people don't continue as vegans are taste, health, and inconvenience (Asher et al. 2014). Let me offer a few recommendations on dealing with former vegans based on the preceding chapters.

We shouldn't insist on "veganissimo" and should avoid thinking in terms of "in" versus "out" or "us" versus "them."
From the Faunalytics study we know that in one-third of cases former vegetarians were living with a non-vegetarian significant other when they began eating animal products again (Asher et al. 2014). As noted, 84 percent of former vegetarians/vegans said they weren't actively involved in a vegetarian/vegan group or organization (potluck, online community, and so on). Clearly, vegetarians and vegans find the support of others invaluable in sticking to their diet. It's incumbent on vegans, therefore, to host potlucks and engage in activism together. As long as a supportive atmosphere exists in these groups, people's resolve will be strengthened.

To tell people that they don't belong because they ate some animal product may spark what psychologists call the "black sheep effect." This is when a member of the in-group is judged more severely and strictly than a member of the out-group (Marques et al. 1988). When a vegan breaks the rules so to speak, others may want to "punish" that individual more severely, either because expectations for that vegan were higher or his or her "fall from grace" is seen as some kind of betrayal, since we thought he or she was "one of us" (remember Daiya cheese?). Whatever the reason, it's bad practice. When people embrace omnivorism, it would be better for vegans to welcome and encourage rather than rebuke them . . . unless we want to be sure we'll never see them again.

We should pay attention to the health pitfalls.

Whether we like it or not, there *are* legitimate health concerns about our diets. If people don't ingest enough vitamin B_{12}, for instance, they can become deficient. The Faunalytics study on former vegetarians shows that 76 percent never had their B_{12} levels checked (Asher et al. 2014). Vegans should insist that new vegetarians or vegans receive all the nutritional information they need, and we should supply trustworthy, evidence-based literature from vegan-registered dieticians.

Ethics are important.

In this book, I suggest that we don't always need to emphasize the moral arguments for not consuming animal products. Moral arguments can meet with resistance, and I've demonstrated that we can drive a lot of change with behavior-first approaches. However, we shouldn't throw the baby out with the bathwater and forget about ethics altogether. Instead, we should recognize its place within a range of options, rather than present-ing veganism as a moral imperative. As stated, I believe that an ethical, ideological approach is likely to be most useful with those already well on their journey to Veganville. Research suggests that an ethical motivation offers people the strongest reason to remain a vegetarian or vegan. More generally, being motivated by more than one reason (health, animals, the environment) seems to encourage people to remain with a vegan diet than only one (Asher et al. 2014, Hoffman et al.).

We need to make veganism even easier.

Much of this book has been about making it easier to become vegan. More reducers will mean greater availability of better products, and an expanded receptivity toward vegetarians and vegans. It's one means of creating a facilitating environment in which reducers and vegetarians can move along the spectrum to veganism, and in which vegans can thrive. That's why everyone concerned with veganism needs to work to deliver more and better alternatives everywhere. We need to create insti-tutional change and change laws and policies. We need to make eating animal products more difficult and expensive. We need to make what is good, easy; and what is easy, the default.

Keeping Activists Active

After fifteen years of leading EVA, I experienced a severe case of burnout. A fellow organizational leader told me: "I can't afford burnout." She felt the animals and her organization needed her to work day and night.

The suffering of animals at human hands is immeasurable. Every second, hundreds of thousands of creatures are abused with a cruelty that is unfathomable, systemic, and utilizes all our ingenuity and technical knowhow. To bear such knowledge and undertake to stop it—especially when virtually everyone around you appears not only indifferent to the suffering but even joyfully complicit in its continuation—is to carry the heaviest of burdens. That's why we need to protect ourselves and work sustainably, not only for ourselves but the animals themselves. Trust me: It's easy to assume as an advocate that you're made of stronger stuff than others, or even to tell yourself that it's better to give the animals five years of maximal effort rather than decades of work at a lesser intensity.

You're wrong on both counts. If I'm any judge, you only think about burnout when it's upon you, which is why I argue that watching out for it should be a permanent, ever-present point of attention for activists. Here are my tips on helping you to keep on keeping on.

It's a marathon, not a sprint.

In the opening chapter, I said that ours is perhaps the hardest struggle ever. That might not sound like much of a motivation, but it should be. Both individually and collectively, the move toward veganism is a big ask, and it's inevitable that it will take time. We shouldn't despair when we don't see change happen fast enough. I don't share the sentiment that we cannot afford to be patient. Actually, I believe we can't afford *not* to be patient. Impatience can burn us out, and when we burn out, the animals have lost an ally. As a movement, we're in this for the long run.

Keep this strategic approach in mind.
The strategy I describe in this book may help make your vegan activism not only more effective but more sustainable. Knowing that every reducer helps make going vegan easier for everyone, and that people don't need to get the animal argument right away (as attitude change may follow behavioral change), might help you to be less impatient and despairing.

It's not just you.
Let's imagine people are like buckets into which compassion needs to be poured. Every time a nonvegan talks to someone, glances over a leaflet, or sees something in the media, more drops are added and the bucket slowly fills. From the outside, we don't know how full that bucket is or how close it is to tipping or overflowing. We may have a general idea of someone's interest, but in my experience it's often the person you least expect who suddenly changes completely. That's a result of hundreds of drops in that bucket over time till it finally overflows. It's important to keep adding, but it's crucial to realize that none of us is responsible on our own for filling anyone else's bucket.

Believe in people.
One criticism leveled at vegans is that they're misanthropic. Unfortunately, in my experience, that is truer than I wish it were. For some vegans to call people the "cancer of the earth" and argue our planet and its nonhuman inhabitants would be better off if we weren't around isn't helpful—not least because they forget that nature is often unpleasant for many animals, with or without our interference.

Although I understand it's hard to take a positive view of humans given our wholesale violence against other species, I nonetheless believe being positive toward our fellow beings is more productive for everyone concerned. I happen to believe that most of us would choose the more humane option if that choice was made easy enough. We can regret that kindness needs to be convenient before most of us will adopt it, but we shouldn't be cynical.

To a certain degree, this book has been about where we, animal advocates, choose to focus our attention. Given a few seconds, most vegans (myself included) could compile a long list of the atrocities people commit. However, what would happen to our outlook if we took some time to add up our species' astonishing achievements, the solutions we've found for problems, or those we admire who are trying to address problems that have so far evaded a solution? At no time in human history have so many been trying to make the planet better for humans or nonhumans. That should be something to build upon.

I believe—much as Stephen Pinker makes the case for the decline in violence over the course of human history—that slowly but surely our societies are moving in the direction of more empathy and rationality, and that both individually and collectively we are becoming more ethical. Whether you share my belief or not, we have a choice on what we focus. Perhaps, as philosopher Karl Popper says, optimism is a moral duty because we can achieve more with a positive mindset. Although some might argue that focusing on the terrible fosters a sense of urgency, I think it can leave us feeling hopeless. Believing in the good may keep us going further and longer.

That's why the governing metaphor of this book—the road to Veganville—works for me: as a journey we've all set out on (occasionally sliding back, but ultimately moving forward). We're each at different stages, some ahead of others. But eventually, all of us will get there.

Don't be (too) angry.
Anger is a powerful, even addictive emotion. We can be angry with animal abusers, those who make money out of animal suffering, feckless politicians, public indifference, or vegans who revert to omnivorism. I understand: The horror is everywhere, and anger salves and energizes.

Yet, although moral outrage has played a significant role in many epochal moments in history, vegans are too few in number for our collective indignation to have a substantial impact. This reality may change someday, but right now we should be careful with our anger. Rage shouldn't be seen

SHOULD WE CONDEMN?

What should vegans do about those who willfully participate in animal cruelty, or mock and belittle any attempts to reduce the consumption of animal products? Given what we know, it's easy for us to condemn everyone who hasn't seen the light.

I'm not a moral relativist: some actions are objectively wrong. However, it's important in our judgments to take into account the times people live in and the pressures of social conformity. (Remember Solomon Asch's experiment?) So much of our society—education, the law, commerce, and other structures—support and encourage thinking and behavior hostile to veganism. Our harshness, therefore, should be tempered by an inquiry into the chances that the individual or group has to think and behave differently. ■

as a sign of one's commitment to the cause, as a prime source of energy and passion, or the fuel that keeps us going. Furthermore, continuous indignation is neither sustainable nor effective in communicating with others. When we're angry, we tend to become judgmental, irrational, hyperbolic, accusatory, adversarial, and see everything as black or white. Would you want to be around such a person?

If we try to walk in other people's shoes, I believe our anger will dissipate. This takes practice, but if you commit to it, it can become habitual. After a while, anger will show up less often and be all the more effective for its rarity. You'll also find it easier to reach out to people and help them.

In the meantime, pummel your pillows, go to the gym, or rant in the privacy of a closed Facebook group or with like-minded friends.

Do something, don't wallow.

It's easy to become paralyzed or depressed by the suffering of animals, or even feel you're obligated to suffer with them. I will admit it's hard to control these feelings of ours, but we can nonetheless make a conscious choice not to wallow in misery. I'm sure the animals would be happier if we were more effective, and being effective requires energy and external focus. If you feel overexposed to atrocities, reframe the narratives: watch or read stories of rescue by shelters and sanctuaries, for instance, rather than dwell on the horrors those animals were saved from.

Be grateful.

Within the misery, we have much to be grateful for. Gratitude feeds instead of drains us. We can be grateful for having the opportunity and means to help and care—something many people can't afford, because of poverty, homelessness, violence, sickness, or political repression. Even our vulnerability can be a source of gratitude. It can motivate us to improve the reality for others.

You're an animal, too!

It's perfectly acceptable to sleep in squats, reject money, and look after five stray dogs—but only by choice. Personal hardship isn't the prerequisite of an effective activist. Professionals with jobs that pay well and offer benefits can be as effective as those who live closer to the edge—probably more so, since a greater degree of material comfort makes an activist life easier to sustain and there's more money to donate. As I argued earlier, it's entirely acceptable to make a living from animal advocacy and veganism—in the private as well as public sectors, as a business owner or a civil-society activist.

You also deserve rest and relaxation. If you can't convince yourself to take a break because the animals need you, tell yourself that you'll be a more effective activist when you're energized and restored. Don't ignore your own happiness. If you love what you do, are good at it, and feel you're making a difference, then your task is to ensure you maintain that feeling. You and the animals deserve no less. ☉

CONCLUSION

The Future of Vegan Strategy and Communication

"The revolution is not a question of virtue, but of effectiveness."
—Jean-Paul Sartre

I have argued in this book that the vegan movement needs a healthy dose of pragmatism. As I write, individuals and society as a whole are too invested in and dependent on animal use for idealistic, moral messages to be sufficient on their own. We have to combine a "Go vegan for the animals" message with "Reduce, for any reason." We need to create a facilitating environment by lobbying and working with the private sector, supporting their efforts to create and market great alternatives to animal products. And we also need to lobby health and environmental NGOs, and the government, to spread awareness and create laws and regulations that facilitate change. Finally, if we want to be more inclusive we may need to relax our concept of veganism.

At some point, the system will change. When that will happen, we don't know. But when it does, it will involve a profound transformation. It won't happen only because of vegans, but because of a high number of reducers. And it won't happen only because of moral awakening, but because of the sustainability and health issues related to animal products, which will increase their price, combined with better and more available alternatives for animal products.

It's my belief that after this tipping point, the need for pragmatism will decrease and the idealistic message will come to the fore. Hearts and minds will be much more receptive to the message of compassion and animal rights. With every new restaurant or store that offers a veggie burger, it becomes easier to approach people with the ethical case for animals. Animal rights advocates will be able to expose speciesist behavior anytime we see it. Direct action and confrontation will be more effective as more will agree with our position. Rescuing animals from factory farms will have more public support. There will be no more need to set the bar low. Veganville will no longer lie atop a distant mountain, but in a nearby valley.

We're not there yet, but I'm entirely confident that we will make it happen. ✪

APPENDIX

Resources

Below are books, blogs, websites, podcasts, and other resources that I recommend, which can help you be a better advocate for animals. Some of these are focused on vegan and animal rights advocacy, others are generic. Anything that doesn't look like a website is a book, for which you'll find the exact reference in the bibliography.

Projects I'm Personally Involved in

- **Veganstrategist.org**: In my own blog, I offer my experiences, thoughts, and tips—sometimes controversial, always thought-provoking—on strategy and communication on a weekly basis. See also facebook.com/veganstrategist.
- **The Center for Effective Vegan Advocacy** (veganadvocacy.org), of which I'm codirector with Melanie Joy. CEVA aims to increase the impact of vegan advocacy worldwide. We give two-day trainings about vegan strategy and communication, all over the world, and also issue grants. CEVA's website also has a resource library for activists. CEVA is a program of Beyond Carnism, an organization dedicated to exposing and transforming carnism, the invisible belief system that conditions people to eat certain animals.
- **ProVeg International** (proveg.com) is a new global food awareness organization I cofounded with Melanie and Sebastian Joy to translate our strategic approach into action. ProVeg's mission is to reduce global animal consumption by 50 percent by 2040. Our vision is a world where everyone chooses delicious and healthy food that is good for all humans, animals, and our planet.

Strategy

- *The Accidental Activist: Stories, Speeches, Articles, and Interviews by Vegan Outreach's Founder*, Matt Ball

- *The Animal Activist's Handbook: Maximizing Our Positive Impact in Today's World*, Matt Ball and Bruce Friedrich
- *Animal Impact: Secrets Proven to Achieve Results and Move the World*, Caryn Ginsberg
- *Changing the Game: Animal Liberation in the Twenty-first Century*, Norm Phelps
- *Made to Stick: Why Some Ideas Take Hold and Others Come Unstuck*, Chip and Dan Heath
- *The Reducetarian Solution: How the Surprisingly Simple Act of Reducing the Amount of Meat in Your Diet Can Transform Your Health and the Planet*, Brian Kateman
- *Strategic Action for Animals: A Handbook on Strategic Movement Building, Organizing, and Activism for Animal Liberation*, Melanie Joy
- *Switch: How to Change Things When Change Is Hard*, Chip and Dan Heath
- *The Tipping Point: How Little Things Can Make a Big Difference*, Malcolm Gladwell
- Veganstrategist.org: my own blog (also on Facebook)

COMMUNICATING AND INFLUENCING MORE EFFECTIVELY
- *How to Win Friends and Influence People*, Dale Carnegie
- *Influence: The Psychology of Persuasion*, Robert Cialdini
- *Nonviolent Communication: A Language of Life*, Marshall Rosenberg
- *Robin Hood Marketing: Stealing Corporate Savvy to Sell Just Causes*, Katya Andreesen

UNDERSTANDING PEOPLE BETTER
- Carnism.org: Carnism explains the psychology of eating animals
- *Change of Heart: What Psychology Can Teach Us about Spreading Social Change*, Nick Cooney
- *Meathooked: The History and Science of Our 2.5-Million-Year Obsession with Meat*, Marta Zaraska

- *The Righteous Mind: Why Good People Are Divided by Politics and Religion*, Jonathan Haidt
- *Some We Love, Some We Hate, Some We Eat: Why It's So Hard to Think Straight about Animals*, Hal Herzog
- *Veganomics: The Surprising Science on What Motivates Vegetarians, from the Breakfast Table to the Bedroom*, Nick Cooney
- *Why We Love Dogs, Eat Pigs and Wear Cows: An Introduction to Carnism*, Melanie Joy

KNOWING WHAT WORKS

- Animalcharityevaluators.org: Effective Altruism–inspired research and recommendations on the most effective animal advocacy organizations
- Faunalytics.org: the world's biggest collection of research about animals
- Mercyforanimals.org/research: studies from Mercy For Animals to improve the effectiveness of farmed-animal advocacy
- Effective Animal Activism: Facebook group with news and discussions on this topic

EFFECTIVE ALTRUISM

- 80000hours.org: career advice for effective altruists
- Effectivealtruism.org: the go-to site for everything EA
- Sentience-politics.org/philosophy: a great primer on the philosophy of Effective Altruism
- *Doing Good Better: Effective Altruism and a Radical New Way to Make a Difference*, William MacAskill
- *How to Be Great at Doing Good: Why Results Are What Counts and How Smart Charity Can Change the World*, Nick Cooney
- *The Most Good You Can Do: How Effective Altruism Is Changing Ideas about Living Ethically*, Peter Singer

Thinking More Clearly and Keeping an Open Mind

- Lesswrong.com: a community blog devoted to redefining the art of human rationality
- Samharris.org/podcast: neuroscientist and philosopher Sam Harris talks with guests about various, often controversial, issues
- *The Art of Thinking Clearly*, Rolf Dobelli

Being Productive and Organized

- *The Seven Habits of Highly Effective People: Powerful Lessons in Personal Change*, Stephen R. Covey
- *Getting Things Done: The Art of Stress-free Productivity*, David Allen
- *Making Ideas Happen: Overcoming the Obstacles between Vision and Reality*, Scott Belsky
- *The Power of Less: The 6 Essential Productivity Principles that Will Change Your Life*, Leo Babauta

Keeping on Keeping on

- Friendly and Pragmatic Vegans and Vegetarians: a Facebook community I recommend
- *The Lifelong Activist: How to Change the World without Losing Your Way*, Hillary Rettig
- *Trauma Stewardship: An Everyday Guide to Caring for Self While Caring for Others*, Laura van Dernoot Lipsky

Staying Healthy and Advocating about Health

- *Becoming Vegan: Comprehensive Edition: The Complete Reference to Plant-based Nutrition*, Brenda Davis and Vesanto Melina
- Jacknorrisrd.com: the blog of vegan dietician Jack Norris
- Nutritionfacts.org, a wealth of vegan nutritional information by Michael Greger, MD
- Theveganrd.com: the blog of vegan dietician Ginny Messina

- *Vegan for Life: Everything You Need to Know to Be Healthy and Fit on a Plant-based Diet*, Jack Norris and Virginia Messina

Business and Entrepreneurship

- Futuremeat.org: the website of the Modern Agriculture Foundation
- GFI.org: the website of the Good Food Institute
- New-harvest.org: New Harvest advances the science behind producing animal products without animals
- *The Personal MBA: A World-class Business Education in a Single Volume*, Josh Kaufman
- Plantbasedfoods.org: the website of the Plant Based Foods Association
- Theplantbasedentrepreneur.com: podcast covering vegan startup founders, business owners, and more

Culinary Education and Advocacy

- Chefchloe.com: Chloe Coscarelli's website, with recipes, videos, books, and other materials
- Foodphotographyschool.com: video course teaching you to take great pictures of your vegan meals
- Naturalgourmetinstitute.com: this New York institute is an established venue for healthy, plant-based cooking
- Plantlab.com: chef and entrepreneur Matthew Kenny's brand, providing plant-based cooking lessons in different countries, and much more
- Rouxbe.com: online cooking classes for both amateurs and professionals, with traditional and plant-based specific content

Specific Topics

- Preventsuffering.org: website of opis, Organisation for the Prevention of Intense Suffering
- Reducing Wild Animal Suffering: Facebook group on this topic

- Vegangmo.com: website that advocates for a rational approach toward biotechnology in the ongoing struggle for animal justice

OTHER RESOURCES

- Colleenpatrickgoudreau.com: podcasts, videos, and blogposts by writer Colleen Patrick-Goudreau
- Mattball.org: the blog of Vegan Outreach cofounder and author Matt Ball
- Unity.fm/program/mainstreetvegan: the podcast of author Victoria Moran
- Medium.com/@TheAnimalist: pragmatic, evidence-based blog about animal advocacy
- Ourhenhouse.org: long-standing podcast about all things vegan and animal rights
- Unnatural Vegan (YouTube): no-nonsense, rational approach to vegan topics
- Vegan.com: the website and the Facebook page, both run by Erik Marcus, contain great stuff. 🌐

Notes

1. Speciesism is the assigning of moral standing and value to an individual (i.e., a human) simply because they belong to a species (i.e. *Homo sapiens*).

2. For an overview of some of the efforts the meat industry makes to keep us committed to eating animal products, and the money they have to do it, see Zaraska, *Meathooked*, chapter 6: "Wagging the Dog of Demand."

3. The term *welfarist* is used pejoratively by part of the animal rights movement to indicate campaigns, messages, or attitudes that are about improving welfare for animals rather than abolishing our use of them.

4. This example is adapted from "Compromise Isn't Complicity," a guest post by Hillary Rettig on my blog, veganstrategist.org, and is based on Adam Hochschild's *Bury the Chains*.

5. It would obviously be wrong to deny that groups of vegans can also have a noticeable and concrete impact on demand. When Tesla brings out cars with a leather-free option, or when the British government considers removing the animal ingredient from their new five-pound notes, they do this for vegans, not for reducers.

6. "Perceived behavioral change" (as opposed to real change) may actually be part of a dissonance reducing strategy (Rothgerber).

7. Of course, one could turn the reasoning around and say that since the meat industry sees through our moderate messaging anyway, we could just as well serve our truth straight up. However, we can assume the general public is not as defensive and suspicious as the meat industry is.

8. I see an interesting paradox in the fact that those who insist that going vegan is exceptionally *easy* are often at the same time the identical people making it appear the *most difficult* by insisting on the highest level of purity.

9. In *Meathooked*, Marta Zaraska explains how similar nationalist and in this case anti-French sentiments were instrumental in taking away Britons' taste for horsemeat (p. 157).

10. Among other elements that influence the attitude–behavior link are the specificity of the attitude, the (perceived) difficulty of the behavior, personality factors such as the degree of self-monitoring, and the strength of the attitude. Regarding the last factor, one study found that participants with a *strong* positive attitude toward Greenpeace were more likely to donate money to the organization one week later. However, attitudes did not predict donation behavior for participants reporting *weak* positive attitudes. Instead, it was their donation behavior that predicted their attitudes toward Greenpeace after they'd had the opportunity to donate or not. For these participants, their attitudes were, thus, shaped by their behavior (Hewstone et al.).

11. For more information about potential benefits of GMO technology, see www.vegangmo.com. ✪

BIBLIOGRAPHY

Abelson, R. P. 1972. "Are Attitudes Necessary?" In B. T. King and E. McGinnies (eds.), *Attitudes, Conflict and Social Change* (New York: Academic Press): 19–32.

Adams, Carol J. 2015. *The Sexual Politics of Meat: A Feminist-Vegetarian Critical Theory: 25th Anniversary Edition* (London: Bloomsbury).

Allen, David. 2001. *Getting Things Done: The Art of Stress-Free Productivity* (London: Penguin).

Alinsky, Saul. 1989. *Rules for Radicals: A Pragmatic Primer for Realistic Radicals* (New York: Vintage).

Andreesen, Katya. 2006. *Robin Hood Marketing: Stealing Corporate Savvy to Sell Just Causes* (San Francisco: Jossey-Bass).

Animal Charity Evaluators. 2015. *Vegetarian Recidivism* <https://animalcharityevaluators.org/research/dietary-impacts/vegetarian-recidivism/>.

Asch, S. E. 1951. "Effects of Group Pressure upon the Modification and Distortion of Judgment." In H. Guetzkow (ed.), *Groups, Leadership and Men* (Pittsburgh: Carnegie Press): 117–90.

——. 1955. "Opinions and Social Pressure," *Scientific American* 193(5): 31–35.

——. 1956. "Studies of Independence and Conformity: I. A Minority of One against a Unanimous Majority," *Psychological Monographs: General and Applied* 70(9): 1–70.

Asher, K., C. Green, H. Gutbrod, M. Jewell, G. Hale, and B. Bastian. 2014. *Study of Current and Former Vegetarians and Vegans: Initial Findings* <https://faunalytics.org/wp-content/uploads/2015/06/Faunalytics_Current-Former-Vegetarians_Full-Report.pdf>.

——. 2016a. *Study of Current and Former Vegetarians and Vegans: Secondary Findings* <https://faunalytics.org/wp-content/uploads/2016/02/Faunalytics-Study-of-Current-and-Former-Vegetarians-and-Vegans--Secondary-Findings-.pdf>.

——. 2016b. *A Summary of Faunalytics Study of Current and Former Vegetarians and Vegans* <https://faunalytics.org/a-summary-of-faunalytics-study-of-current-and-former-vegetarians-and-vegans/>.

Babauta, Leo. 2009. *The Power of Less: The 6 Essential Productivity Principles that Will Change Your Life* (Carlsbad, Calif.: Hay House).

Ball, Matt. 2014. *The Accidental Activist: Stories, Speeches, Articles, and Interviews by Vegan Outreach's Founder* (New York: Lantern).

Ball, Matt, and Bruce Friedrich. 2009. *The Animal Activist's Handbook: Maximizing Our Positive Impact in Today's World.* (New York: Lantern).

Bandura, A. 1977. "*Self-efficacy: Toward a Unifying Theory of Behavioral Change,*" *Psychological Review* 84(2): 191–215.

Beardsworth, A., and T. Keil. 1997. *Sociology on the Menu: An Invitation to the Study of Food and Society* (London: Routledge).

Belsky, Scott. 2011. *Making Ideas Happen: Overcoming the Obstacles between Vision and Reality* (London: Penguin).

Berscheid, E. 1966. "Opinion Change and Communicator–Communicatee Similarity and Dissimilarity," *Journal of Personality and Social Psychology* 4: 670–80.

Bird, Susan. 2016. *Vegan Butcher Opens Doors and the Meat Industry Goes Nuts,* Care2.com <http://www.care2.com/causes/vegan-butcher-opens-doors-and-the-meat-industry-goes-nuts.html>.

Bolotsky, Josh. n.d. *Use Your Radical Fringe to Shift the Overton Window,* Beautiful Trouble n.d. <http://beautifultrouble.org/principle/use-your-radical-fringe-to-shift-the-overton-window/>.

Brennan, L., and W. Binney. 2010. "Fear, Guilt, and Shame Appeals in Social Marketing," *Journal of Business Research* 63(2): 140–46.

Carnegie, Dale. 2006/1936. *How to Win Friends and Influence People* (London: Random House).

Choi, Candice. 2015. "End of Meat? Startups Seek Meat Alternatives for the Masses," The Big Story (AP), December 29 <http://bigstory.ap.org/article/c3d68aac0b094faf9273ddefff67cf7e/end-meat-startups-seek-alternatives-masses>.

Cialdini, Robert. 2007/1984. *Influence: The Psychology of Persuasion* (New York: Collins Business).

Cialdini, R., J. Demaine, B. Sagarin, D. Barrett, K. Rhoads, and L. Winter. 2006. "Managing Social Norms for Persuasive Impact," *Social Influence* 1(1): 3–15.

Coetzee, J. M. 2003. *Elizabeth Costello* (London: Penguin).

Cooney, Nick. 2011. *Change of Heart. What Psychology Can Teach Us about Spreading Social Change* (New York: Lantern).

———. 2014. *Veganomics: The Surprising Science on What Motivates Vegetarians from the Breakfast Table to the Bedroom* (New York: Lantern).

———. 2015. *How to Be Great at Doing Good: Why Results Are What Counts and How Smart Charity Can Change the World* (San Francisco: Jossey-Bass).

Covey, Stephen. 1989. *The Seven Habits of Highly Effective People: Powerful Lessons in Personal Change* (New York: Fireside).

Cuddy, Amy. 2015. *Presence: Bringing Your Boldest Self to Your Biggest Challenges* (New York: Little, Brown).

Costello, K., and G. Hodson. 2010. "Exploring the Roots of Dehumanization: The Role of Animal–Human Similarity in Promoting Immigrant Humanization," in *Group Processes & Intergroup Relations* 13: 3–22.

———. 2014. "Lay Beliefs about the Causes of and Solutions to Dehumanization and Prejudice: Do Non-experts Recognize the Role of Human–Animal Relations?" *Journal of Applied Social Psychology* 44: 278–88.

Davis, Brenda, and Vesanto Melina. 2014. *Becoming Vegan: Comprehensive Edition. The Complete Reference to Plant-based Nutrition* (Summertown, Tenn.: Book Publishing Company).

Dhont, K., and G. Hodson. 2014. "Why Do Right-wing Adherents Engage in More Animal Exploitation and Meat Consumption?" *Personality and Individual Differences* 64: 12–17.

———. 2015. "The Person-based Nature of Prejudice: Individual Difference Predictors of Intergroup Negativity," *European Review of Social Psychology* 26: 1–42.

Dhont, K., G. Hodson, and A. C. Leite. 2016. "Common Ideological Roots of Speciesism and Generalized Ethnic Prejudice: The Social Dominance Human–Animal Relations Model" (SD–HARM), *European Journal of Personality* 30: 507–22.

Dobelli, Rolf. 2013. *The Art of Thinking Clearly* (London: Hodder & Stoughton).

Duhigg, Charles. 2012. *The Power of Habit: Why We Do What We Do and How to Change.* (London: Random House).

Eagly, A. H. 1978. "Sex Differences in Influenceability," *Psychological Bulletin* 85: 86–116.

Faunalytics. 2007. *Advocating Meat Reduction and Vegetarianism to Adults in the US* <https://faunalytics.org/wp-content/uploads/2016/02/HRC-Veg-Study-2007-Full-Report-HRC-MASTER.pdf>.

———. 2012. *Why or Why Not Vegetarian?* <http://faunalytics.org/wp-content/uploads/2015/05/Fundamentals_Why-Why-Not-Vegetarian.pdf>.

Ferriss, Tim. 2016. "Ezra Klein: From College Blogger to Political Powerhouse," <http://tim.blog/2016/12/13/ezra-klein/> December 12.

Festinger, L. 1957. *A Theory of Cognitive Dissonance* (Stanford: Stanford University Press).

Fhaner, G., and M. Hane. 1979. "Seat Belts: Opinion Effects of Law-induced Use," *Journal of Applied Psychology* 64: 205–12.

Fiddes, Nick. 1991. *Meat: A Natural Symbol* (London: Routledge).

Freedman, J., and S. Fraser. 1966. "Compliance without Pressure: The Foot-in-the-door Technique," *Journal of Personality and Social Psychology* 4: 195–203.

Gladwell, Malcolm. 2000. *The Tipping Point: How Little Things Can Make a Big Difference* (New York: Back Bay).

Godin, Seth. 2015. "How Idea Adoption Works: The Idea Progression," Seth Godin's website, September <http://sethgodin.typepad.com/seths_blog/2015/09/how-idea-adoption-works-the-idea-progression.html>.

———. 2017. "The Two Vocabularies (Because There Are Two Audiences)," Seth Godin's website, February <http://sethgodin.typepad.com/seths_blog/2017/02/the-two-vocabularies-because-there-are-two-audiences.html>.

Ginsberg, Caryn. 2011. *Animal Impact: Secrets Proven to Achieve Results and Move the World* (Arlington, Va.: Priority Ventures).

Haidt, Jonathan. 2013. *The Righteous Mind: Why Good People Are Divided by Politics and Religion* (New York: Vintage).

Haines, H. 2013. "Radical Flank Effects," in D. Snow, D. della Porta, B. Klandermans, and D. McAdam (eds.), *The Wiley Blackwell Encyclopedia of Social and Political Movements* (Chichester, Eng.: Wiley Blackwell).

Hamilton, M. 2006. "Eating Death: Vegetarians, Meat and Violence," *Food, Culture & Society* 9(2): 155–77.

Harrison-Dunn, Annie-Rose. 2014. "Brits Moving to Non-dairy Pastures: Mintel Report," <http://www.foodnavigator.com/Market-Trends/Dairy-alternatives-on-the-up-Mintel>.

Haverstock K., and D. Forgays. 2012. "To Eat or Not to Eat: A Comparison of Current and Former Animal Product Limiters," *Appetite* 58: 1030–36.

Heath, Chip, and Dan Heath. 2008. *Made to Stick: Why Some Ideas Take Hold and Others Come Unstuck* (London: Arrow).

———. 2010. *Switch: How to Change Things When Change Is Hard* (London: Random House).

Herzog, Hal. 2011. *Some We Love, Some We Hate, Some We Eat: Why It's So Hard to Think Straight about Animals* (New York: Harper Perennial).

Hewstone, M., W. Stroebe, and K. Jonas. 2012. *An Introduction to Social Psychology: Fifth Edition* (Oxford: Blackwell).

Hochschild, Adam. 2006. *Bury the Chains: Prophets and Rebels in the Fight to Free an Empire's Slaves* (New York: Mariner).

Hoffman, S., S. Stallings, R. Bessinger, and G. Brooks. 2013. "Differences between Health and Ethical Vegetarians: Strength of Conviction, Nutrition Knowledge, Dietary Restriction, and Duration of Adherence," *Appetite* 65: 139–44.

Holland, R., B. Verplanken, and A. Van Knippenberg. 2002. "On the Nature of Attitude-behavior Relations: The Strong Guide, The Weak Follow," *European Journal of Social Psychology* 32(6): 869–76.

Humane League Labs. 2014. "Diet Change and Demographic Characteristics of Vegans, Vegetarians, Semi-vegetarians, and Omnivores" <http://www.humaneleaguelabs.org/blog/2014-04-07-large-scale-survey-vegans-vegetarians-and-meat-reducers/>.

Interlandi, Jeneen. 2015. "The Brain's Empathy Gap: Can Mapping Neural Pathways Help Us Make Friends with Our Enemies?" *New York Times*, March 19.

Ivox research, commissioned by EVA. 2016. Research among 1,000 Flemish people.

IVU (International Vegetarian Union). n. d. "The Vegetarian World Forum" 1(5) (Spring 1951): 6–7 <http://www.ivu.org/history/world-forum/1951vegan.html>.

Joy, Melanie. 2008. *Strategic Action for Animals: A Handbook on Strategic Movement Building, Organizing, and Activism for Animal Liberation* (New York: Lantern).

———. 2010. *Why We Love Dogs, Eat Pigs and Wear Cows: An Introduction to Carnism* (San Francisco: Conari Press).

Kateman, Brian. 2017. *The Reducetarian Solution: How the Surprisingly Simple Act of Reducing the Amount of Meat in Your Diet Can Transform Your Health and the Planet* (New York: Tarcher Perigee).

Kaufman, Josh. 2012. *The Personal MBA: A World-class Business Education in a Single Volume* (London: Penguin).

Knowles, E. S., and J. A. Linn. 2004. *Resistance and Persuasion* (Mahwah, N.J.: Erlbaum).

Kolbert, Elizabeth. 2017. "Why Facts Don't Change Our Minds. New Discoveries about the Human Mind Show the Limitation of Reason," *New Yorker*, February 27.

Kraus, S. 1995. "Attitudes and the Prediction of Behavior: A Meta-analysis of the Empirical Literature," *Personality and Social Psychology Bulletin* 21(1): 58–75.

Kreausukon, P., P. Gellert, S. Lippke, and R. Schwarzer. 2012. "Planning and Self-efficacy Can Increase Fruit and Vegetable Consumption: A Randomized Controlled Trial," *Journal of Behavioral Medicine* 35(4): 443–51.

Lea, E., and A. Worsley. 2003. "Benefits and Barriers to the Consumption of a Vegetarian Diet in Australia," *Public Health Nutrition* 6(5): 505–11.

Leenaert, Tobias. 2017. "When Activists Mean Business: An Interview with David Benzaquen," Vegan Strategist, February 8 <http://veganstrategist.org/2017/02/08/business-is-not-a-four-letter-word-an-interview-with-david-benzaquen/>.

———. 2016. "The Extremely Inconvenient Truth of Wild Animal Suffering," Vegan Strategist, June 1 < http://veganstrategist.org/2016/06/01/the-extremely-inconvenient-truth-of-wild-animal-suffering/>.

Levitt, T. 2011. "Jonathan Safran Foer: Environmentalists Who Eat Meat Have a Blind Spot," *The Ecologist*," January 24 <http://www.theecologist.org/Interviews/739796/jonathan_safran_foer_environmentalists_who_eat_meat_have_a_blindspot.html>.

Loughnan S., N. Haslam, and B. Bastian. 2010. "The Role of Meat Consumption in the Denial of Moral Status and Mind to Meat Animals," *Appetite* 55(1): 156–59.

McEwen, Annie and Matt Kielty. 2016. "Alpha Gal," Radiolab, October 27 <radiolab.org/story/alpha-gal>.

MacAskill, William. 2016. *Doing Good Better: Effective Altruism and a Radical New Way to Make a Difference* (New York: Penguin).

Marques, J., V. Yzerbyt, and J-P Leyens. 1988. "The "Black Sheep Effect": Extremity of Judgments towards Ingroup Members as a Function of Group Identification," *European Journal of Social Psychology* 18(1): 1–16.

Maurer, Donna. 2012. *Vegetarianism: Movement or Moment?* (Philadelphia: Temple University Press).

Meindertsma, Christien. 2010. "How Pig Parts Make the World Turn," TEDtalk <https://www.youtube.com/watch?v=BRETz2F-heQ>.

Messina, Virginia. 2015. "Preventing Ex-Vegans: Why Feeling 'Normal' Matters," VeganRD, July <http://www.theveganrd.com/2015/07/preventing-ex-vegans-why-feeling-normal-matters.html>.

Meyers, David G. 2011. *Psychology: Tenth Edition* (New York: Worth Publishers).

Minson, Julia A., and Benoît Monin. 2012. "Do-Gooder Derogation: Disparaging Morally Motivated Minorities to Defuse Anticipated Reproach," *Social Psychological and Personality Science* 3(2) 2012: 200–7.

Mullee, A., L. Vermeire, B. Vanaelst, B. et al. "Vegetarianism and Meat Consumption: A Comparison of Attitudes and Beliefs between Vegetarian, Semi-vegetarian, and Omnivorous Subjects in Belgium. *Appetite* forthcoming.

Nibert, David. 2002. *Animal Rights/Human Rights: Entanglements of Oppression and Liberation* (Lanham, Md.: Rowman & Littlefield).

Norris, Jack, and Virginia Messina. 2011. *Vegan for Life: Everything You Need to Know to Be Healthy and Fit on a Plant-based Diet* (Boston: Da Capo).

Our Hen House. 2016. "The Good Food Institute's Bruce Friedrich and a Review of Vegan Everyday Stories from Eric Milano and Laura Delhauer," July, episode 338 <http://www.ourhenhouse.org/2016/07/episode-338-the-good-food-institutes-bruce-friedrich-and-a-review-of-vegan-everyday-stories-from-eric-milano-and-laura-delhauer>.

Phelps, Norm. 2015. *Changing the Game: Animal Liberation in the Twenty-first Century* (New York: Lantern).

Piazza J., M. B. Ruby, S. Loughnan, M. Luong, J. Kulik, H. M. Watkins, and M. Seigerman. 2015. "Rationalizing Meat Consumption. The 4Ns," *Appetite* 91: 114–28.

Piazza, J., and S. Loughnan. 2016. "When Meat Gets Personal, Animals' Minds Matter Less: Motivated Use of Intelligence Information in Judgments of Moral Standing," *Social Psychological and Personality Science* 7(8): 876–84.

Pinker, Stephen. 2011. *The Better Angels of Our Nature: A History of Violence and Humanity* (London: Penguin).

Potts, Annie. 2010. "Vegan Sexuality: Challenging Heteronormative Masculinity through Meat-free Sex," in *Feminism & Psychology* 20: 53–72.

Purdy, Chase. 2016. "Inside the Battle to Convince America to Eat Meatless Burgers," *Quartz*, December 11 <https://qz.com/853332/behind-the-fight-to-convince-people-to-buy-meatless-burgers/>.

Regan, Tom. 2004/1983. *The Case for Animal Rights* (Oakland: University of California Press).

Rettig, Hillary. 2006. *The Lifelong Activist: How to Change the World without Losing Your Way* (New York: Lantern).

——. 2016. "Compromise Isn't Complicity," Vegan Strategist, November 6 <http://veganstrategist.org/2015/11/06/compromise-isnt-complicity-four-reasons-vegan-activists-should-welcome-reducetarianism-and-one-big-reason-reducetarians-should-go-vegan/>.

Reuter, T., J. P. Ziegelmann, A. U. Wiedemann, C. Geiser, S. Lippke, B. Schüz, B., and R. Schwarzer. 2010. "Changes in Intentions, Planning, and Self-efficacy Predict Changes in Behaviors: An Application of Latent True Change Modeling," *Journal of Health Psychology* 15: 935–47.

Robbins, James. 1992. "How Capitalism Saved the Whales," Foundation for Economic Education <https://fee.org/articles/how-capitalism-saved-the-whales/>.

Rogers, Everett M. 2003. *Diffusion of Innovations: Fourth Edition*. New York: Free Press.

Rosenberg, Marshall. 2003. *Nonviolent Communication: A Language of Life* (Encinitas, Calif.: Puddledancer Press).

Rothgerber, Hank. 2014. "Efforts to Overcome Vegetarian-induced Dissonance among Meat Eaters," *Appetite* 79: 33.

Schwitzgebel, E. 2013. "The Moral Behaviour of Ethics Professors and the Role of the Philosopher," Schwitzsplinters.com, September 3, 2013 <http://schwitzsplinters.blogspot.co.uk/2013/09/the-moral-behavior-of-ethics-professors.html>.

Schwitzgebel E., and J. Rust. 2014. "The Moral Behavior of Ethics Professors: Relationships among Self-reported Behavior, Expressed Normative Attitude, and Directly Observed Behaviour," *Philosophical Psychology* 27(3): 1–35.

Serpell, James. 1996. *In the Company of Animals: A Study of Human–Animal Relationships* (Cambridge: Cambridge University Press).

Sethu, Harish. 2015. "How Many Animals Does a Vegetarian Save?" Counting Animals, March 16 <http://www.countinganimals.com/how-many-animals-does-a-vegetarian-save/>.

Shore, Randy. 2015. "B.C. Companies Thrive as Meatless Eating Goes Mainstream," *Vancouver Sun*, November 20 <http://www.vancouversun.com/health/companies+thrive+meatless+eating+goes+mainstream/11550063/story.html>.

Singer, Peter. 1995. *Animal Liberation: Second Edition* (London: Pimlico).

———. 1998. *Ethics into Action: Henry Spira and the Animal Rights Movement* (Lanham, Md.: Rowman & Littlefield).

———. 2015. *The Most Good You Can Do: How Effective Altruism is Changing Ideas about Living Ethically* (New Haven: Yale University Press).

Spiegel, Marjorie. 1989. *The Dreaded Comparison: Human and Animal Slavery* (New York: Mirror Books).

Thaler, Richard, and Cass Sunstein. 2009. *Nudge: Improving Decisions about Health, Wealth and Happiness* (London: Penguin).

Thomson, Lars, and Reuben Proctor. 2013. *Veganissimo A to Z: A Comprehensive Guide to Identifying and Avoiding Ingredients of Animal Origin in Everyday Products* (New York: The Experiment).

Tuttle, Stacey. 2013. "Lincoln Movie—Thoughts on a Compass," Shepherd Project, February 21 <http://shepherdproject.com/lincoln-thoughts-on-a-compass/>.

Van Dernoot Lipsky, Linda. 2009. *Trauma Stewardship: An Everyday Guide to Caring for Self While Caring for Others* (San Francisco: Berrett-Koehler).

Van Zomeren, M., T. Postmes, and R. Spears. 2008. "Toward an Integrative Social Identity Model of Collective Action: A Quantitative Research Synthesis of Three Socio-psychological Perspectives," *Psychological Bulletin* 134: 504–35.

Vegan Bros. n.d. "Say This to Convince a Hunter to Go Vegan" <http://veganbros.com/hunters-go-vegan/>.

VRG. 2016. "How Many People Are Vegetarian or Vegan?" Vegetarian Resource Group <http://www.vrg.org/nutshell/faq.htm#poll>.

Wansink B., and J. Kim. 2005. "Bad popcorn in Big Buckets: Portion Size Can Influence Intake as Much as Taste," *Journal of Nutrition Education and Behavior* 37(5): 242–45.

Wicker, A. 1969. "Attitude Versus Actions: The Relationship of Verbal and Overt Behavioral Responses to Attitude Objects," *Journal of Social Issues* 25(4): 41–78.

Williams, Daren. 2012. "What's Wrong with Meatless Monday?" Beltway Beef, February 16 <https://beltwaybeef.wordpress.com/category/meatless-monday/>.

Williams, Nancy. 2008. "Affected Ignorance and Animal Suffering: Why Our Failure to Debate Factory Farming Puts Us at Moral Risk," *Journal of Agricultural and Environmental Ethics* 21(4): 371–84.

Winslow, Gren. 2015. "Dropping in on the Animal Rights Movement," Canadian Cattlemen, October 19 <http://www.canadiancattlemen.ca/2015/10/19/dropping-in-on-the-animal-rights-movement/>.

Zane D., J. Irwin, and R. Walker Reczek. 2015. "Do Less Ethical Consumers Denigrate More Ethical Consumers? The Effect of Willful Ignorance on Judgments of Others," *Journal of Consumer Psychology* 26(3): 337–49.

Zaraska, Marta. 2016. *Meathooked: The History and Science of Our 2.5-Million-Year Obsession with Meat* (New York: Basic). ☮

ACKNOWLEDGMENTS

Like many animal advocates interested in strategy, throughout the years I've taken part in many online and offline discussions and debates about what works, what works better, and what doesn't. I've also read countless articles, blogposts, and books by many people. I'm bound to forget many of the people that I am indebted to for shaping my thinking, but here is an attempt to name some of them:

Lyra Alves, Matt Ball, Martin Balluch, Brock Bastian, Vincent Berraud, Carolina Bertolaso, Jon Bockman, Lewis Bollard, Maarten Boudry, Stijn Bruers, Wolf Bullman, Angela Carstensen, Chen Cohen, Nick Cooney, Hans Dagevos, Jasmijn De Boo, Helen Duke, John Edmundson, Joe Espinoza, Lucie Evers, Joanne Fairbrother, Bernie Fischlowitz-Roberts, Swayze Foster, Rebecca Fox, Dan Friedman, Bruce Friedrich, Moritz Friedrich, Sarah Gilroy, Caryn Ginsberg, Matthew Glover, Dobrusia Gogloza, Che Green, Lisa Green, Zach Groff, Gabi Helfert, Alex Hershaft, Wayne Hsiung, Louis Jans, Brian Kateman, Andrew Kirschner, Jonathan Leighton, Matt and Phil Letten, Axel Lieber, Jeffrey Lins, Christine Lofgren, Jo-Anne McArthur, Adriano Mannino, Jesse Marks, Ricardo Marques, Eisel Mazard, Suzanne McMillan, Kristina Mering, Pablo Moleman, Mikael Nielsen, Sharon Nuñez, David Olivier, Fouke Ombelet, Heather Patrick, David Pearce, David Pedersen, Kurt Peleman, Jared Piazza, Jacy Reese, Hillary Rettig, Luc Rombaut, Jeff Rosenberg, Hank Rothgerber, Stijn Scholts, Harish Sethu, Paul Shapiro, Allison Smith, Charles Stahler, Kim Stallwood, Eva Supply, Brett Thompson, Seth Tibbott, Brian Tomasik, Gabriele Vaitkevičiūtė, Jose Valle, Wannes Van Giel, Patrick Van Wynsberghe, Michel Vandenbosch, Pieter Vanderwegen, Jef Vervoort, Elaine Vigneault, Jeroen Willemsen, and all my former colleagues at EVA. I'm also indebted to the work of Dale Carnegie, Jonathan Haidt, Chip and Dan Heath, Erik Marcus, Colleen Patrick-Goudreau, Norm Phelps, Tom Regan, Peter Singer, and many others.

Special thanks again go to Peter Singer for writing the foreword and for being a lifelong inspiration; to Amy Hall-Bailey for the cover design and illustrations; to Kathryn Asher, Margaret Chandler, Kristof Dhont, Melanie Joy, Sebastian Joy, Alex Lockwood, and Jens Tuider for their thorough comments on the manuscript. My publisher Martin Rowe at Lantern Books has been an incredible help with his meticulous editing and knowledge about the issues. I'm also especially grateful to my partner and fellow activist Melanie Jaecques and our pack of canines and felines for supporting me.

Finally, a huge thank you also to you for reading this book and for everything you do to make this world a better place for all sentient beings. 🌐

About the Author

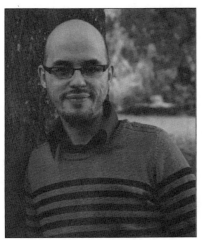

Tobias Leenaert is a longtime speaker, trainer, and strategist. He is also the cofounder and former director of the Belgian organization EVA (Ethical Vegetarian Alternative), the first vegetarian/vegan organization to receive structural funding from a national government. Under Tobias' management, EVA launched a successful campaign that resulted with the city of Ghent becoming the first city ever to officially support a weekly vegetarian day. Tobias gives animal advocacy trainings worldwide together with Melanie Joy, for the Center of Effective Vegan Advocacy (CEVA). He is also cofounder of ProVeg International, a new international pro-vegan food awareness organization with the mission to reduce the global consumption of animals by 50 percent by the year 2040. Tobias lives in Ghent, Belgium, with his partner, two dogs, and six cats. He blogs at www.veganstrategist.org and welcomes your thoughts at tobias@veganstrategist.org.

ABOUT THE PUBLISHER

LANTERN BOOKS was founded in 1999 on the principle of living with a greater depth and commitment to the preservation of the natural world. In addition to publishing books on animal advocacy, vegetarianism, religion, and environmentalism, Lantern is dedicated to printing books in the U.S. on recycled paper and saving resources in day-to-day operations. Lantern is honored to be a recipient of the highest standard in environmentally responsible publishing from the Green Press Initiative.

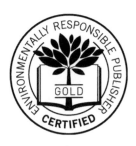

lanternbooks.com